Immunotherapy for Head and Neck Cancer

头颈部肿瘤的免疫治疗

原　著　陈德章（Anthony T. C. Chan）
　　　　马碧如（Brigette B. Y. Ma）
主　审　王俊杰　李宝生
主　译　田素青　茅芯慧　韩　光

北京大学医学出版社

TOUJINGBU ZHONGLIU DE MIANYI ZHILIAO

图书在版编目（CIP）数据

头颈部肿瘤的免疫治疗 / 陈德章, 马碧如原著; 田素青, 茅芯慧, 韩光主译. -- 北京: 北京大学医学出版社, 2025. 3. -- ISBN 978-7-5659-3345-5

Ⅰ. R739.915.1

中国国家版本馆 CIP 数据核字第 2024H4D225 号

北京市版权局著作权合同登记号：图字：01-2024-6259

First published in English under the title
Immunotherapy for Head and Neck Cancer
edited by Anthony T.C. Chan and Buig Yue Brigette Ma
Copyright © Anthony T.C. Chan and Buig Yue Brigette Ma, under exclusive license to Springer Nature Switzerland AG, 2023
This edition has been translated and published under licence from Springer Nature Switzerland AG.

Simplified Chinese translation Copyright © 2025 by Peking University Medical Press.
All Rights Reserved.

头颈部肿瘤的免疫治疗

主　　译：	田素青　茅芯慧　韩　光
出版发行：	北京大学医学出版社
地　　址：	（100191）北京市海淀区学院路 38 号　北京大学医学部院内
电　　话：	发行部 010-82802230；图书邮购 010-82802495
网　　址：	http://www.pumpress.com.cn
E－mail：	booksale@bjmu.edu.cn
印　　刷：	中煤（北京）印务有限公司
经　　销：	新华书店
责任编辑：张凌凌	责任校对：靳新强　责任印制：李　啸
开　　本：	710 mm × 1000 mm　1/16　印张：12　字数：180 千字
版　　次：	2025 年 3 月第 1 版　2025 年 3 月第 1 次印刷
书　　号：	ISBN 978-7-5659-3345-5
定　　价：	88.00 元

版权所有，违者必究

（凡属质量问题请与本社发行部联系退换）

译者名单

（按姓名汉语拼音排序）

韩　光　湖北省肿瘤医院

雷润宏　北京大学第三医院

李　涛　北京大学第三医院

刘　伟　北京大学第三医院

鲁　瑛　湖北省肿瘤医院

茅芯慧　新疆维吾尔自治区人民医院

田素青　北京大学第三医院

肖　宇　北京大学第三医院

许　璐　宜昌市中心人民医院

易廷庄　右江民族医学院附属医院

余笑言　湖北省肿瘤医院

袁　程　宜昌市中心人民医院

周亚娟　湖北省肿瘤医院

序一

免疫治疗作为一种颠覆传统的新兴治疗方式，正在为医学界开辟新的治疗模式，为患者带来更多选择与希望。本书凝聚了头颈部肿瘤免疫治疗领域近年来的重要研究成果，既包括头颈部肿瘤免疫治疗的基础概念、理论、机制，又重点关注研究进展和临床应用，多角度展现了头颈部肿瘤免疫治疗的现状与未来研究方向，兼具全面性与系统性，条理清晰，实用性强，能为读者提供相关指导或实践参考。

作为一名长期致力于肿瘤治疗研究的学者，我希望本书能为国内同行提供帮助，为推动肿瘤研究与临床实践贡献力量。同时，也期待它能激发更多探索与创新，为患者的健康带来更多福祉。

中国工程院院士　于金明

2025 年 1 月

序二

得知《头颈部肿瘤的免疫治疗》一书即将出版，我非常高兴，本书是 Immunotherapy for Head and Neck Cancer 一书的中文翻译版，而我本人恰好也是英文版原著的作者之一，所以对这本书的内容非常了解。

近年来，免疫治疗作为一种新兴的肿瘤治疗手段，受到了越来越多的关注。尤其在头颈部肿瘤治疗领域，免疫治疗展现出巨大的潜力和价值，为患者带来了新的希望。如何更好地将理论与临床相结合，是当前面临的重要课题。本书对头颈部肿瘤免疫治疗基础和临床方面重要的科学研究文献进行了全面的汇总，内容涵盖了基础理论、最新研究进展和临床应用现状，为研究人员和临床医生提供了一本系统而实用的参考书。

本书的翻译引进离不开译者团队的努力，他们认真翻译、仔细审校，忠实地呈现了原著的精髓，为国内读者深入了解头颈部肿瘤免疫治疗的前沿动态提供了便利，有助于为未来的研究和应用开拓新视野。

希望本书能够为国内同仁带来帮助，希望大家一起努力，在未来的研究和实践中，找到更多适合中国患者的治疗方案，为患者带来更多希望。

中国科学院院士　马骏
2025 年 1 月

译者前言

在头颈部肿瘤治疗领域，免疫治疗近年来快速发展，免疫检查点抑制剂和其他免疫治疗策略的应用已逐渐改变了患者的治疗模式和预后。为了能与广大同行共同了解、学习头颈部肿瘤免疫治疗领域的最新研究成果，我们组织翻译了《头颈部肿瘤的免疫治疗》一书，旨在为读者提供一本内容全面、方便随时查阅的实用参考书。

本书内容包括丰富的基础研究、临床试验数据，以及真实世界的治疗经验，深入探讨了免疫治疗在头颈部肿瘤治疗中的潜力与挑战。作为译者，我们在翻译过程中力求准确传达原著的学术精髓，同时也特别关注本书内容的可读性与医学专业性，以便于读者更好地理解和应用这些先进的免疫治疗理念。由于原著含有大量的英文专业术语的缩写，为了方便读者查阅与理解，我们在中文版的最后专门附上了专业术语缩略语表。

头颈部肿瘤的免疫治疗是一个前沿且充满挑战的领域，是全球范围内肿瘤学研究的热点之一。希望通过这本书，能为相关专业人员提供宝贵的参考资料，推动国内这一领域的进一步发展。

感谢原作者的辛勤工作，也感谢每一位为此书付出努力的人。希望本书能够为广大的医学读者群体提供一个深入理解和探讨肿瘤免疫治疗的新视角，助力更好的临床实践，惠及患者福祉。

田素青
2024 年 12 月

目 录

引言 1
Introduction

第 1 章　头颈部肿瘤的免疫学：免疫逃逸机制与肿瘤微环境 5
Immunological Landscape of Head and Neck Cancer: Mechanisms of Immune Escape and the Tumor Microenvironment

第 2 章　头颈部肿瘤免疫治疗临床开发中的药物靶点与策略 25
Drug Targets and Strategies in the Clinical Development of Immunotherapy for Head and Neck Cancer

第 3 章　免疫治疗在局部晚期鼻咽癌中的应用 53
Immunotherapy in Locally Advanced Nasopharyngeal Carcinoma

第 4 章　免疫治疗在复发 / 转移性鼻咽癌中的应用 65
Immunotherapy in Recurrent and Metastatic Nasopharyngeal Carcinoma

第 5 章　超越 PD-1/PD-L1 免疫检查点抑制剂：头颈部肿瘤的其他靶点与治疗方法 75
Beyond PD-1/PD-L1 Immune Checkpoint Inhibitors: Other Targets and Approaches for Head and Neck Cancer

第 6 章　免疫治疗联合放疗在头颈部肿瘤中的转化与临床研究 99
Translational and Clinical Approach to Combining Immunotherapy with Radiotherapy in the Treatment of Head and Neck Cancer

第 7 章　免疫治疗在头颈部肿瘤围术期管理中的临床应用 119
Clinical Application of Immunotherapy in the Perioperative Management of Head and Neck Cancer

第 8 章　免疫检查点抑制剂在罕见头颈部肿瘤治疗中的作用 143
The Role of Immune Checkpoint Inhibitors in the Treatment of Less Common Head and Neck Cancers

第 9 章　头颈部肿瘤免疫治疗预测生物标志物的发展 157
Development of Predictive Biomarkers to Immunotherapy in Head and Neck Cancer

专业术语缩略语表 171

引言

Introduction

头颈部肿瘤（head and neck cancer, HNC）是一组在流行病学、生物学和治疗方面异质性极强的肿瘤。总体而言，2021年，因口腔癌、喉癌、鼻咽癌、口咽癌、下咽癌和涎腺癌而死亡的人数共467 125人，占同年990万癌症相关死亡的4.7%[1]。头颈部鳞状细胞癌（squamous cell cancer of the head and neck, HNSCC）*是全球最常见的头颈部肿瘤亚型，其传统治疗方法包括手术治疗、放射治疗（简称放疗）和化学治疗（简称化疗）。长期以来，对于没有治愈性治疗选择的复发/转移性（recurrent/metastatic, R/M）HNSCC患者，治疗选择主要限于化疗。免疫治疗（immunotherapy, IO）直到2006年才被视为HNSCC的"主流"治疗方法，当时针对表皮生长因子受体（epidermal growth factor receptor, EGFR）的嵌合型单克隆抗体西妥昔单抗被批准用于治疗接受过铂类药物治疗的R/M HNSCC患者，作为单药治疗，以及与放疗联合用于治疗局部晚期HNSCC[2-3]。西妥昔单抗是第一种与以铂类药物为基础的化疗（简称铂类化疗）联用时能够延长生存期的免疫治疗药物（西妥昔单抗与铂类化疗联用即所谓的EXTREME方案），在R/M HNSCC的一线治疗中使用[4]。然而，从2006年开始的免疫治疗的兴起很快就结束了，直到10年后，当第一个针对免疫检查点蛋白程序性死

---

*译者注：在部分英文文献中头颈部鳞状细胞癌也被称为squamous cell carcinoma of the head and neck，缩写为SCCHN，为避免歧义，本书统一使用HNSCC作为头颈部鳞状细胞癌的英文缩写。

亡受体 1（programmed cell death receptor 1，PD-1）的抗体纳武利尤单抗（nivolumab）2016 年在 CHECKMATE-141 研究中被批准用于治疗铂类药物难治性 R/M HNSCC 患者，头颈部肿瘤免疫治疗的"黄金时期"才真正开始 [5]。此后，R/M HNSCC 患者的中位生存期从以往单纯使用铂类化疗的不足 6 个月，提高到与 EXTREME 方案联用的超过 10 个月，再到 KEYNOTE-048 研究中将帕博利珠单抗添加到铂类化疗后的几乎达到 15 个月 [6]。在 R/M 非角化鼻咽癌（一种在中国南部和东南亚流行的与 Epstein-Barr 病毒相关的 HNC）中也可以观察到免疫治疗对患者生存的影响。这场免疫治疗的复兴改变了 HNC 的治疗范式。目前正在进行数百项新的临床试验，这些试验以免疫检查点抗体为治疗主干，在各种临床环境中用于 HNC 治疗。

本书是关于头颈部鳞状细胞癌、鼻咽癌（nasopharyngeal cancer，NPC）以及其他较少见的头颈肿瘤（如涎腺癌）免疫治疗的科学研究亮点汇编。本书有多学科作者团队，各作者均为各自领域的领军人物，在本书的 9 个章节中，他们详细介绍了 HNC 免疫治疗的最新进展。本书内容回顾了从实验室到临床的发展历程，从 HNC 免疫逃逸机制的概述开始，接着简要总结了在姑息性治疗、根治性治疗和新辅助治疗中免疫治疗和生物标志物的临床开发。在本书中概述的科学成就证明了那些未放弃寻找更好 HNC 治疗方法的人的价值，他们包括参与免疫治疗临床试验的患者，以及敢于挑战常规并推动临床进步的研究者。

我们衷心感谢所有不顾全球新型冠状病毒大流行带来的挑战而辛勤工作的本书贡献者。我们希望感谢为本项工作提供支持的 Alice Kong 女士。我们还要感谢李氏慈善基金会，该基金会通过香港中文大学的精准免疫治疗计划对本项工作提供了部分支持。

参考文献

1. Sung H, Ferlay J, Siegel RL et al (2021) Global cancer statistics 2020: GLOBOCAN estimates of incidence and mortality worldwide for 36 cancers in 185 countries. CA Cancer J Clin 71(3):209–249. doi: https://doi.org/10.3322/caac.21660
2. Bonner JA, Harari PM, Giralt J et al (2006) Radiotherapy plus cetuximab for squamous-cell carcinoma of the head and neck. N Engl J Med 354(6):567–578. doi: https://doi.org/10.1056/NEJMoa053422
3. Bonner JA, Harari PM, Giralt J et al (2010) Radiotherapy plus cetuximab for locoregionally advanced head and neck cancer: 5-year survival data from a phase 3 randomised trial, and relation between cetuximab-induced rash and survival. Lancet Oncol 11(1):21–28. doi: https://doi.org/10.1016/S1470-2045(09)70311-0
4. Vermorken JB, Mesia R, Rivera F et al (2008) Platinum-based chemotherapy plus cetuximab in head and neck cancer. N Engl J Med 359(11):1116–1127. doi: https://doi.org/10.1056/NEJMoa0802656
5. Ferris RL, Blumenschein G Jr, Fayette J et al (2016) Nivolumab for recurrent squamous-cell carcinoma of the head and neck. N Engl J Med 375:1856–1867. doi: https://doi.org/10.1056/NEJMoa1602252
6. Burtness B, Harrington KJ, Greil R et al (2019) Pembrolizumab alone or with chemotherapy versus cetuximab with chemotherapy for recurrent or metastatic squamous cell carcinoma of the head and neck (KEYNOTE-048): a randomised, open-label, phase 3 study. Lancet 394(10212):1915–1928. doi: https://doi.org/10.1016/S0140-6736(19)32591-7

马碧如（Brigette B. Y. Ma）
陈德章（Anthony T. C. Chan）

State Key Laboratory of Translational Oncology,
Department of Clinical Oncology, Sir YK Pao
Centre for Cancer, Hong Kong Cancer Institute,
The Charlie Lee Precision Immunotherapy Program
The Chinese University of Hong Kong,
Shatin, Hong Kong SAR

第1章 头颈部肿瘤的免疫学：免疫逃逸机制与肿瘤微环境

Immunological Landscape of Head and Neck Cancer: Mechanisms of Immune Escape and the Tumor Microenvironment

（Nicole C. Schmitt, Brendan L. C. Kinney, Robert L. Ferris 著）
（田素青，茅芯慧 译）

摘要

为了形成肿瘤，转化细胞必须从免疫系统的持续压力中逃逸出来。肿瘤细胞内部和肿瘤微环境组成的变化包括几种免疫逃逸机制。尽管头颈部肿瘤的肿瘤突变负荷相对较高，但它们常存在抗原处理机制的缺陷，从而削弱了新生抗原向免疫细胞呈递的能力。免疫效应细胞可能数量稀少，功能耗竭，或者被肿瘤微环境中的免疫抑制细胞、免疫抑制细胞因子、趋化因子所抑制。尽管抗肿瘤免疫功能障碍在人乳头瘤病毒（human papillomavirus，HPV）阴性的头颈部肿瘤中尤为显著，但由HPV驱动的肿瘤也能够通过独特的免疫逃逸机制实现免疫逃逸。

原作者信息

N.C. Schmitt (✉) · B. L. C. Kinney
Winship Cancer Institute at Emory University School of Medicine, Atlanta, GA, USA
e-mail: nicole.cherie.schmitt@emory.edu

R. L. Ferris
University of Pittsburgh School of Medicine, UPMC Hillman Cancer Center, Pittsburgh, PA, USA
e-mail: ferrrl@upmc.edu

> **关键词**
>
> 抗原加工机制·头颈部肿瘤·人乳头瘤病毒·免疫逃逸·髓源性抑制细胞·调节性 T 细胞

1　引言

抗肿瘤免疫反应的发生依赖于多个关键环节。其中至关重要的是肿瘤必须被免疫细胞识别为外来或转化的细胞。在先天性免疫反应中，自然杀伤细胞（natural killer cell，NK 细胞）通过识别并清除表面表达异常或应激信号的肿瘤细胞来发挥作用，这些信号包括细胞表面主要组织相容性复合体（major histocompatibility complex，MHC）表达水平的降低（图 1-1）。T 细胞对肿瘤细胞的识别依赖于肿瘤抗原的表达。这类抗原可以是突变多肽（如突变型 p53）或病毒致癌蛋白（如 HPV 相关蛋白）。肿瘤相关抗原（tumor-associated antigen，TAA）是指（与正常细胞相比）在肿瘤细胞中异常高表达的蛋白质，例如表皮生长因子受体（growth factor receptor，EGFR）。为了使这些抗原被免疫细胞识别，它们必须经过抗原加工并通过 MHC 呈递至细胞表面（图 1-2）。免疫细胞，尤其是 CD8+ 细胞毒性 T 细胞（cytotoxic T lymphocyte，CTL），需要在肿瘤微环境中存在并被充分激活，才能对这些肿瘤抗原产生效应性反应。若上述任何一个环节出现缺失或功能异常，抗肿瘤免疫反应将变得低效或完全丧失。此外，免疫抑制细胞（如髓源性抑制细胞和调节性 T 细胞）及免疫抑制细胞因子的存在，会削弱 CTL 在肿瘤微环境中的迁移能力及对转化上皮细胞的杀伤能力。头颈部肿瘤涉及多种免疫逃逸机制，本章将对这些机制进行详细探讨。

2　免疫编辑与肿瘤突变负荷

如前所述，适应性抗肿瘤免疫反应的关键在于对肿瘤新生抗原

第 1 章 头颈部肿瘤的免疫学：免疫逃逸机制与肿瘤微环境

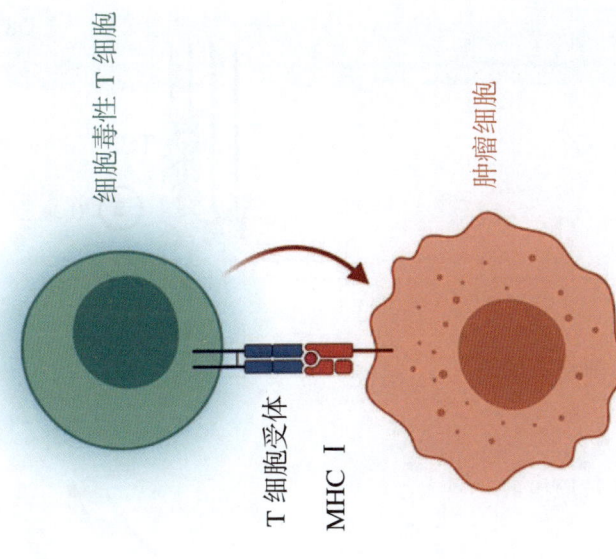

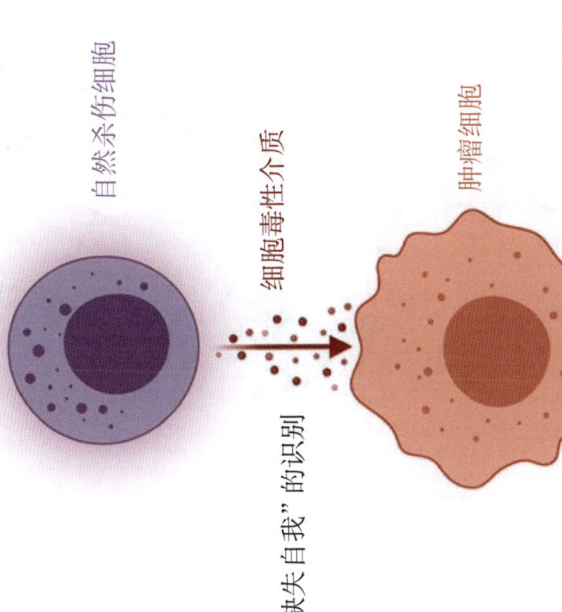

图 1-1 先天性和适应性抗肿瘤免疫反应。自然杀伤细胞（NK 细胞）通过检测细胞表面缺乏 MHC I 表达的细胞来识别异常细胞，并释放细胞毒性分子。适应性免疫反应依赖于识别 MHC I 呈递的肿瘤抗原，然后由抗原特异性 T 细胞受体（T cell receptor，TCR）识别。本图通过 Biorender.com 绘制。

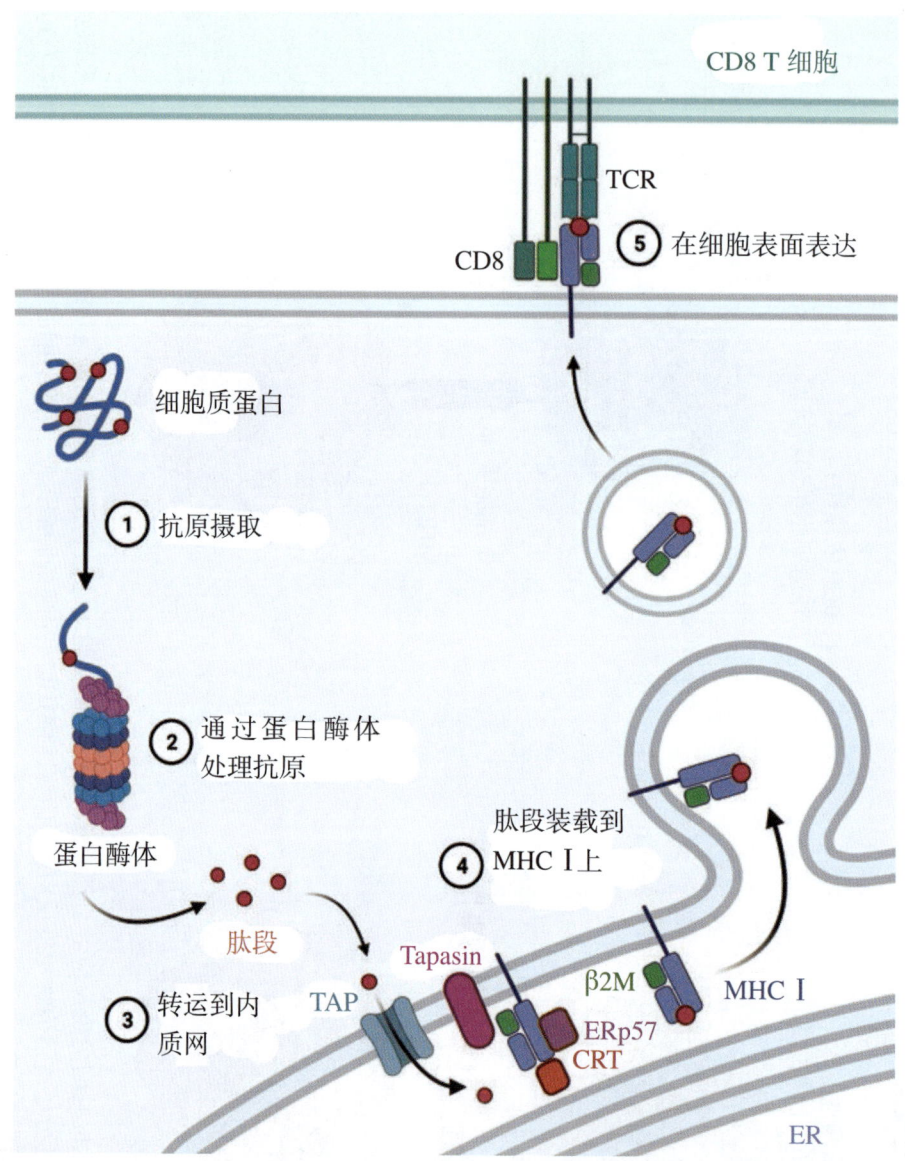

图 1-2　抗原加工与呈递需要一系列步骤。首先，细胞质蛋白通过蛋白酶体被处理成肽段，然后通过抗原加工相关转运蛋白（transporter associated with antigen processing, TAP）被转运到内质网。接着，一系列伴侣蛋白帮助 MHC Ⅰ 进行折叠 / 组装以及抗原肽装载。MHC- 抗原复合物随后被运输到细胞表面，以呈递给抗原特异性 T 细胞受体（TCR）。本图通过 Biorender.com 绘制。

(neoantigen)的有效识别。尽管某些肿瘤突变的免疫原性显著高于其他突变，但肿瘤突变负荷（tumor mutational burden, TMB）高的肿瘤通常伴随更高的免疫效应细胞浸润，并对免疫治疗表现出更显著的治疗反应[1]。事实上，免疫监视（immunosurveillance）过程能够在很大程度上防止转化细胞和突变细胞发展为肿瘤[2]。然而，随着时间推移，肿瘤可能通过诱导T细胞对病毒致癌蛋白或突变肽产生耐受性，从而逃避免疫系统对新生抗原的识别[3]。在持续的免疫压力下，肿瘤逐渐演化出逃逸亚群，这些亚群的肿瘤细胞可能丧失新生抗原表达或丧失其他能够被T细胞和NK细胞识别的关键因子[2]。这一过程被称为免疫编辑（immunoediting），它通常分为三个阶段（图1-3）：清除、平衡、逃逸。①清除阶段（elimination phase）：在此阶段，转化细胞被先天性免疫细胞（如NK细胞）和适应性免疫细胞（如细胞毒性T细胞）识别并清除。②平衡阶段（equilibrium phase）：部分转化细胞逃脱清除，并在免疫压力下进入静止状态，与免疫系统处于动态平衡。③逃逸阶段（escape phase）：由于免疫系统的持续抑制作用，转化细胞逐渐扩增，突破免疫控制，最终形成肿瘤。在逃逸阶段，除了新生抗原表达丧失外，还有其他免疫逃逸机制发挥作用，包括：免疫效应细胞的功能障碍或缺失，抗原加工和呈递机制的异常，免疫检查点的抑制信号与共刺激信号之间的失衡，肿瘤微环境中免疫抑制细胞及免疫抑制细胞因子的富集。这些免疫逃逸机制在头颈部肿瘤中的具体表现及其临床意义将在本章后续部分中深入探讨。

3 抗原加工元件

抗原加工元件（Antigen Processing Machinery, APM）是一组酶类和分子伴侣，它们负责生成抗原表位并将其转运至内质网（endoplasmic reticulum, ER），以及将MHC Ⅰ[MHC也称人类白细胞抗原（human leukocyte antigen, HLA）]正确折叠并使其与β2-微球蛋白（beta-2-microglobulin，β2M）结合，随后将抗原装载到MHC Ⅰ上，再通过细胞表面呈递给免疫细胞（图1-2）。上述过程始于刺激蛋白酶体转化

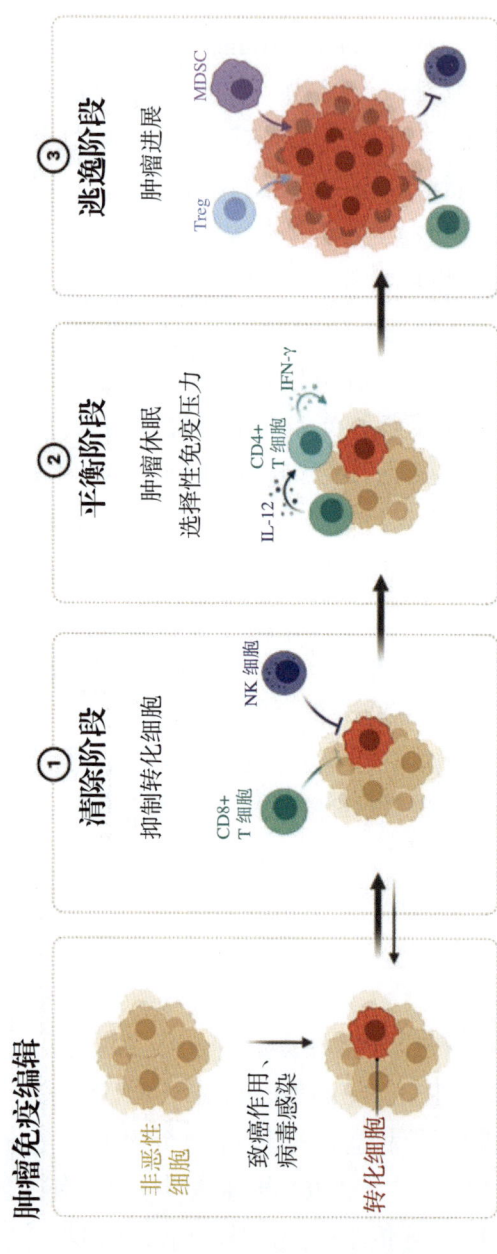

图 1-3 肿瘤免疫编辑的过程需要三个主要步骤（三个阶段）：清除、平衡和逃逸。在清除阶段，转化细胞被免疫效应细胞抑制或消灭。为抵抗免疫压力，转化细胞进行适应性调整，进入平衡状态。最后，转化细胞内部或微环境中进一步的适应性改变使这些细胞从免疫压力中逃逸出来，从而使它们迅速分裂并形成肿瘤。NK 细胞：自然杀伤细胞；IL-12：白介素 12；IFN-γ：干扰素 γ；Treg：调节性 T 细胞；MDSC：髓源性抑制细胞。本图通过 Biorender.com 绘制。

为免疫蛋白酶体，该转化通过用低分子量蛋白（low molecular weight protein，LMP）2、7、10（即 LMP2、LMP7、LMP10）取代蛋白酶体的 β1、β2、β5 亚基来实现[4-7]。含有 LMP2、LMP7、LMP10 的免疫蛋白酶体能够生成具有适当大小并与 MHC Ⅰ 结合槽具有高亲和力的抗原[4]。这些抗原表位经过降解后，由 TAP1 和 TAP2 组成的异二聚体转运至内质网腔[4-7]。在内质网腔内，抗原肽通过内质网氨肽酶 1 和 2（即 ERAP1 和 ERAP2）的进一步加工，达到 8~11 个氨基酸的理想长度。随后，在分子伴侣钙网蛋白（calreticulin）、钙连接蛋白（calnexin）、ERp57 和 TAP 相关蛋白（TAP-associated protein，Tapasin）的协助下，抗原（antigen，Ag）被装载并稳定于 MHC Ⅰ 重链 -β2M 轻链聚合物的结合槽内[4-7]。稳定的 Ag-MHC Ⅰ -β2M 三聚体最终通过高尔基体转运至细胞表面，供免疫细胞识别[4-7]。这一通路的正常功能对于细胞毒性 T 细胞（CTL）识别并清除恶性细胞至关重要[7-9]。

大多数 APM 组分的表达主要通过由干扰素 γ（interferon gamma，IFN-γ）介导的信号通路调控，其中关键的信号分子包括 JAK2（Janus kinase 2，Janus 激酶 2）和 STAT1（signal transduer and activator of transcription 1，信号转导及转录激活因子 1）[4-12]。IFN-γ 通过两个途径促进 LMP2 和 LMP7（从而促进蛋白酶体向免疫蛋白酶体的转化）、TAP1、TAP2、Tapasin、HLA Ⅰ 和 β2M 的表达：一是通过 JAK/STAT 磷酸化级联反应，产生能够与上述 APM 组分启动子区域的 γ 活化序列（gamma-activated sequence，GAS）结合的磷酸化 STAT1（pSTAT1）同源二聚体[7]；二是通过核蛋白 NLRC5 的表达与激活，NLRC5 是 NOD 样受体家族含半胱天冬酶募集结构域的蛋白 5（NOD-like receptor family, caspase recruitment domain containing 5），又称 Ⅰ 类转录激活因子（class Ⅰ transactivator, C Ⅰ TA）[11]。除了 IFN-γ 途径外，TAP1 的表达还可以通过 p53 和 p73 独立或协同诱导，这种反应模式通常发生在 DNA 损伤时[11]。这种冗余机制的重要性已通过体外实验得到证明：将 TAP1 的 cDNA 转染到肿瘤细胞系中，结果表明单独增加 TAP1 的表达就足以诱导 CTL 对先前逃避免疫清除的细胞的识别和清除[9]。

头颈部鳞状细胞癌（HNSCC）中遗传学改变的证据较少[5]，但除此之外，HNSCC 中 MHC/HLA Ⅰ 及其他 APM 相关基因的遗传学改变非常普遍。在原发性 HNSCC 病灶中，约有 15% 的病例存在 HLA Ⅰ 基因的完全丢失，37% 的病例则为选择性丢失，这些改变导致功能异常[4-5]。虽然 MHC Ⅰ 的缺失可能使肿瘤细胞更易被 NK 细胞杀死，但这些改变却严重削弱了转化细胞激活适应性（抗原特异性）免疫反应的能力。导致 APM 功能障碍的主要原因是上游转录因子的调控失常[10]，尤其是 STAT1 的异常。在 HNSCC 中，pSTAT1 的基础水平显著降低，这与表皮生长因子受体（EGFR）的过表达密切相关。EGFR 的过表达引发含 Src 同源结构域的磷酸酶 2（Src homology domain-containing phosphatase 2, SHP2）的异常表达[8]。研究表明，SHP2 能够主动去磷酸化 pSTAT1，从而减少 IFN-γ 诱导的 APM 组分的表达[8]。此外，SHP2 的过表达还通过下调 RANTES 和 IP10 介导免疫抑制肿瘤微环境的形成[8]。目前关于 NLRC5 失调的研究比较少，因为它是近期发现的分子。然而，有研究表明，在约 20% 的 HNSCC 病灶中，NLRC5 存在拷贝数丢失[11]。关于 TAP1 的表达调控，还需考虑 p53 的改变。功能性 p53 的缺失会削弱细胞在应对 DNA 损伤时通过上调 TAP1 实现冗余表达的能力[12]。

APM 多个组分的表达水平与患者的生存预后密切相关。除 HLA Ⅰ 的下调外，Tapasin 的下调与上颌窦鳞状细胞癌患者的生存率下降也存在关联；此外，LMP2、LMP7、TAP1、TAP2 以及 HLA Ⅰ 的表达降低与头颈部不同解剖部位肿瘤的生存率呈负相关[5, 10]。一项研究发现，在该研究分析的头颈部肿瘤中，80% 的病例至少有一个 APM 组分出现下调[10]。这构成了一个累积效应问题，因为任何一个 APM 组分的下调都会导致功能性 Ag-HLA Ⅰ -β2M 三聚体的表面呈递不足[10]。HLA Ⅰ 表面呈递不足会削弱 CTL 清除恶性细胞的能力[4-9]，进而导致许多本应有效的疗法（如免疫检查点阻断疗法）在 APM 能力受损的恶性肿瘤中疗效不佳。

4　免疫效应细胞

当头颈部肿瘤细胞既无法有效表达和呈递抗原，也未能产生足够的损伤相关分子模式（damage-associated molecular pattern，DAMP）以诱导炎症和激活先天性免疫反应时，肿瘤微环境中募集的免疫效应细胞会极为稀少。这种免疫"冷"肿瘤（immunologically cold tumor）通常与较差的临床预后和对免疫治疗的低响应率相关。相比之下，免疫"热"肿瘤（immunologically hot tumor）因具有大量免疫效应细胞浸润，通常表现出更好的免疫治疗反应（图1-4）。通过整合基因组分析，HPV阴性头颈部肿瘤被分为几个亚型：经典型（classical type）、基底型（basal type）和炎性/间质型（inflamed/mesenchymal type）。其中炎性/间质型的抗原呈递相关基因及辅助性T细胞（T-helper cell）分化相关基因皆为高表达[13]。同样，HPV驱动的肿瘤也可以被分为经典型和炎性/间质型[13]，这部分解释了为何某些"冷型"HPV阳性肿瘤预后较差。本章后续部分将详细讨论HPV驱动的头颈部肿瘤特有的免疫逃逸机制。

免疫效应细胞不仅需要存在于肿瘤微环境中，还必须保持功能活性，才能发挥有效的抗肿瘤免疫作用。然而，某些治疗方式可能严重影响免疫效应细胞的功能。例如，高剂量铂类化疗显著抑制T细胞的增殖和细胞因子分泌[14]；反复的低剂量放疗也可能对免疫效应细胞产生类似的免疫抑制效应[15]。此外，免疫检查点分子的表达会显著削弱免疫效应细胞的功能，从而限制抗肿瘤免疫反应的效果。

5　免疫检查点

共抑制检查点（co-inhibitory checkpoint）包括程序性死亡受体1（PD-1）和细胞毒性T淋巴细胞相关抗原4（cytotoxic T lymphocyte-associated antigen 4，CTLA-4）等，在免疫系统中的作用是抑制过度免疫反应（如自身免疫）。然而，在长期暴露于病毒感染或肿瘤抗原的情况下，T细胞会逐渐上调抑制性检查点分子的表达，导致其进入功能性"耗竭"状态。这一状态使T细胞无法有效发挥抗肿瘤免疫作用。尽

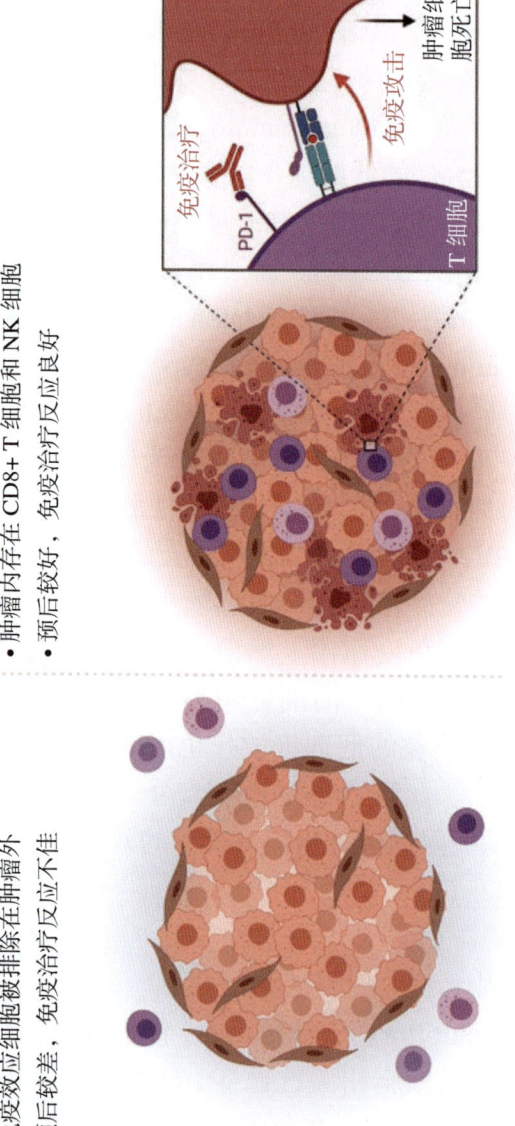

图 1-4 与免疫"热"肿瘤相比,缺乏免疫效应细胞的免疫"冷"肿瘤与预后不良和对免疫治疗反应差相关。本图通过 Biorender.com 绘制。

管 PD-1 和 CTLA-4 是目前研究最深入的共抑制检查点，其他分子如 T 细胞免疫球蛋白黏蛋白 3（T cell immunoglobulin mucin-3, TIM-3）和淋巴细胞活化基因 3（lymphocyte activation gene-3, LAG-3）也在头颈部肿瘤的发生发展中起重要作用[3]。与此同时，T 细胞的共刺激受体（co-stimulatory receptor），如 CD27、CD28、CD137 和 OX40，其表达水平可能下降，而这些受体对维持 T 细胞的最佳功能至关重要[16-17]。T 细胞的功能在很大程度上取决于共抑制检查点和共刺激检查点间的动态平衡。例如，在头颈部肿瘤中，丧失共刺激受体 CD27 和 CD28 表达的 T 细胞被发现新获得了 PD-1 和 TIM-3 的表达，这些 T 细胞进入功能失调状态，并对其他 T 细胞产生抑制作用[17]。作为一种免疫治疗策略，靶向共抑制检查点和（或）共刺激检查点已成为治疗头颈部肿瘤的研究热点，本书其他章节将对此类免疫治疗策略展开更详细的讨论。

6　免疫抑制细胞与免疫抑制细胞因子

免疫效应细胞的功能可由共抑制检查点和共刺激检查点的平衡决定，与此类似，肿瘤微环境的影响主要取决于免疫刺激细胞及免疫刺激细胞因子与免疫抑制细胞及免疫抑制细胞因子间的动态平衡（图 1-5）。肿瘤微环境中的细胞因子可分为以下两类：第一类（免疫刺激型）：包括干扰素 -γ（IFN-γ）、白介素 2（IL-2）和白介素 12（IL-12），能够促进效应 T 细胞的功能；第二类（免疫抑制型）：包括白介素 4（IL-4）、白介素 6（IL-6）、白介素 10（IL-10），对 T 细胞功能具有抑制作用。免疫抑制细胞因子、生长因子和趋化因子，如转化生长因子 β（transforming growth factor beta, TGF-β）、IL-6、IL-10、粒细胞 - 巨噬细胞集落刺激因子（granulocyte-macrophage colony-stimulating factor, GM-CSF）和前列腺素 E2（prostaglandin E2, PGE2），可由肿瘤细胞及免疫抑制细胞分泌，进一步调节肿瘤微环境[18-20]。

髓源性抑制细胞（myeloid-derived suppressor cell, MDSC）是一类未成熟的髓系细胞，正常情况下以低水平存在于外周血，并在生理条

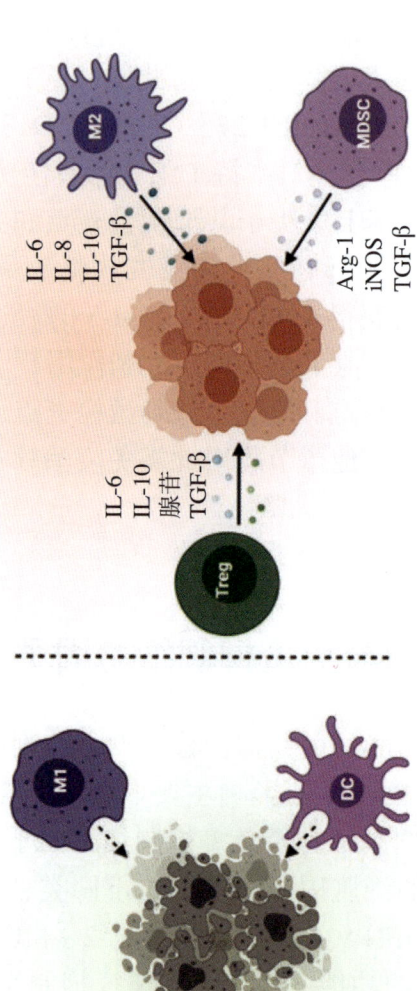

图 1-5 肿瘤微环境中的免疫刺激细胞包括自然杀伤（NK）细胞、细胞毒性 T 细胞（CTL）、M1 型巨噬细胞和树突细胞（dendritic cell, DC）。M1 型巨噬细胞和 DC 可以吞噬肿瘤细胞碎片。免疫抑制细胞包括 M2 型巨噬细胞、髓源性抑制细胞（MDSC）和调节性 T 细胞（Treg），它们分泌促肿瘤的细胞因子和代谢物。本图通过 Biorender.com 绘制。

件下分化为巨噬细胞、中性粒细胞或树突细胞。然而，在肿瘤患者中，MDSC 可能在血液中大量累积，并迁移至肿瘤微环境，在局部发挥免疫抑制作用。MDSC 包括两种主要亚型：单核型 MDSC（monocytic MDSC, M-MDSC）和多形核型 MDSC（polymorphonuclear MDSC, PMN-MDSC），两者在功能和表面标志物上有所不同。这些 MDSC 可通过 GM-CSF、MCP-1、CXCL1、IL-8 和 CSF1 等细胞因子和趋化因子被募集至肿瘤微环境[21]，也在肿瘤微环境中由其他单核细胞转化而来。一旦在肿瘤内聚集，MDSC 就会分泌精氨酸酶 1（arginase-1）、一氧化氮合酶和活性氧（reactive oxygen species, ROS）等物质，这些物质通过直接损害或消耗代谢资源抑制效应 T 细胞的功能[21]。研究表明，从头颈部肿瘤患者中分离的 MDSC 以 STAT3 依赖性方式产生精氨酸酶 1，并显著抑制 T 细胞增殖[22]。此外，PMN-MDSC 的高水平与头颈部肿瘤的晚期阶段和较差的生存预后密切相关[23-24]。

肿瘤相关巨噬细胞（tumor-associated macrophage, TAM）在肿瘤微环境中表现出两种主要表型：M1 型与 M2 型。M1 型（免疫刺激型）具有促炎和抗肿瘤特性；M2 型（免疫抑制型）通过分泌免疫抑制细胞因子（如 TGF-β、IL-6、IL-8、IL-10）以及精氨酸酶 1 抑制 T 细胞和 NK 细胞的功能[21]。在头颈部肿瘤中，M2 型巨噬细胞较为常见，其丰度与肿瘤的转移潜能及不良生存预后显著相关[25]。与巨噬细胞类似，CD4+ 辅助性 T 细胞可以分化为两个亚型：TH1 型（免疫刺激型）和 TH2 型（免疫抑制型）。

调节性 T 细胞（regulatory T cell, Treg）是免疫抑制细胞的重要亚群。Treg 是 CD4+ T 细胞的一种亚型，同时表达 Foxp3、CD25 和 CTLA-4。Treg 既可以通过趋化因子被募集至肿瘤微环境，也可以由未分化的 CD4+ T 细胞在肿瘤微环境中分化生成。进入肿瘤后，Treg 可以通过分泌免疫抑制细胞因子（如 TGF-β 和 IL-10）发挥免疫抑制功能，还可通过分泌穿孔素和颗粒酶直接杀伤效应性免疫细胞[21, 26]。此外，Treg 表面的 CD39 可将 ATP 转化为腺苷，进一步抑制免疫反应[27]。Treg 表面的 CTLA-4 与树突细胞的 CD80/CD86 结合，减少 CD28 与 CD80/CD86 的结合机会，从而限制 T 细胞的共刺激信号，进一步削弱免疫活性[21]。尽管 Treg 在多种肿瘤中被认为促进免疫逃逸，但在头颈部肿瘤中，

Treg 的预后意义仍存在争议 [21, 28-30]，说明 Treg 对头颈部肿瘤免疫环境的影响可能比之前认为的更复杂。

7　HPV 驱动疾病的特殊免疫逃逸机制

当前，大多数口咽鳞状细胞癌（oropharyngeal squamous cell carcinoma, OPSCC）由人乳头瘤病毒（HPV）的慢性感染驱动。为了在口咽区域持续感染并诱发恶变，HPV 必须首先成功逃避宿主的抗病毒免疫反应。研究表明，免疫抑制状态（如人类免疫缺陷病毒感染、先天性免疫缺陷、自身免疫性疾病以及器官移植后的医源性免疫抑制）与 HPV 驱动恶性肿瘤的高发病率密切相关 [31]。此外，在 HPV 相关 OPSCC 中，较高水平的肿瘤浸润性淋巴细胞（tumor-infiltrating lymphocyte, TIL）通常与更好的预后相关 [32]。这表明免疫功能障碍是 HPV 相关癌症发病的关键因素。

HPV 拥有高度策略性的生命周期，使其能够有效逃避宿主的免疫监视。病毒感染始于基底细胞上皮层，该区域的免疫细胞密度较高，但病毒的早期基因产物表达水平非常有限。在这一阶段，病毒通过低水平的 E6 和 E7 致癌蛋白表达维持其隐匿性，病毒 DNA 以附加体（episome）的形式整合于宿主细胞中 [33]。随着宿主细胞分化为成熟的角质形成细胞并迁移至上皮表面（该区域免疫细胞数量显著减少），病毒的复制及 E6/E7 的表达显著增加。衣壳蛋白（HPV 的高度免疫原性成分）仅在角质形成细胞脱落前生成，从而大幅限制了抗原暴露于免疫系统的机会 [34]。此外，HPV 通过随宿主上皮细胞的自然脱落而释放，而不需要宿主细胞裂解，从而避免了通常会引发免疫反应的炎症信号 [34-38]。

HPV 的致癌蛋白（特别是 E6 和 E7）通过多种途径抑制宿主的先天性和适应性免疫反应。例如，研究表明，E6 和 E7 可以抑制干扰素及其相关基因的生成，而这些基因对于启动强有力的抗肿瘤免疫反应至关重要 [31, 33-34, 36, 39-40]。此外，约 20% 的 HPV 驱动 OPSCC 病例中存在肿瘤坏死因子受体相关因子 3（TNF receptor-associated factor 3, TRAF-3）的失活突变，该基因在病毒感染期间的干扰素生成及 NF-κB 信号通路的激活中发挥重要作用[41]。HPV 的 E6 和 E7 蛋白还可通过下调 Toll 样受体 9（Toll-like receptor 9，TLR9）的表达进一步削弱免疫系统的抗病毒能力[42-43]。此外，HPV 致癌蛋白能够抑制抗原加工元件（APM）的多个关键组分，包括 TAP1、TAP2、Tapasin、MHC Ⅰ 和 MHC Ⅱ 以及 LMP2[34, 36, 42, 44-46]。HPV 阳性肿瘤中还常观察到大量的调节性 T 细胞浸润以及功能失调或耗竭的 CD8+ T 细胞，这进一步削弱了抗肿瘤免疫反应[47-48]。

关于免疫检查点在 HPV 阳性和 HPV 阴性 HNSCC 中的作用，目前尚存争议，在 HPV 阳性和 HPV 阴性 HNSCC 中 PD-1/PD-L1 表达的研究结果也并不一致[49]。一项将 TIL 中 PD-1 的表达水平分为低、中、高三类的研究发现 HPV 阳性肿瘤的 TIL 更可能表现为 PD-1 阳性，然而，PD-1 高表达的 TIL 在 HPV 阴性肿瘤中更为常见，并且与更差的生存预后相关[49]。

8　结论

转化细胞为了形成肿瘤并茁壮成长，必须绕过或克服几层免疫压力。在近几十年中，我们对肿瘤细胞和肿瘤微环境逃避免疫监视和免疫杀伤的策略有了更多了解。对这些免疫逃逸机制的深入理解已经促使研究者设计出几种不同的抗肿瘤免疫治疗方法。随着我们进一步理解免疫逃逸的机制，这些免疫治疗策略可能会继续扩展和改进。

原文符合伦理标准相关声明

Conflicts of Interest　NCS has received research funding for Astex Pharmaceuticals and has done consulting for Checkpoint Surgical. RLF has the following disclosures:

Achilles Therapeutics: Advisory Board.
Aduro Biotech, Inc.: Consulting.
Astra-Zeneca/MedImmune: Clinical Trial, Research Funding.
Bicara Therapeutics, Inc.: Consultant.
Bristol-Myers Squibb: Advisory Board, Clinical Trial, Research Funding.
EMD Serono: Advisory Board.
Everest Clinical Research Corporation: Consultant.

F. Hoffmann-La Roche Ltd.: Consultant.
Genocea Biosciences, Inc.: Consultant.
Instil Bio, Inc.: Advisory Board.
Kowa Research Institute, Inc.: Consultant.
Lifescience Dynamics Limited: Advisory Board.
MacroGenics, Inc.: Advisory Board.
Merck: Advisory Board, Clinical Trial.
Mirati Therapeutics, Inc.: Consultant.
Nanobiotix: Consultant.
Novasenta: Consulting, Stock, Research Funding.
Numab Therapeutics AG: Advisory Board.
OncoCyte Corporation: Advisory Board.
Pfizer: Advisory Board.
PPD: Consultant.
Rakuten Medical, Inc.: Advisory Board.
Sanofi: Consultant.
Seagen, Inc.: Advisory Board.
Tesaro: Research Funding.
Zymeworks, Inc.: Consultant.

Funding Supported in part by Winship Cancer Institute of Emory University.

参考文献

1. Mandal R, Samstein RM, Lee KW et al (2019) Genetic diversity of tumors with mismatch repair deficiency influences anti-PD-1 immunotherapy response. Science 364:485-491. https://doi.org/10.1126/science.aau0447
2. Dunn GP, Ikeda H, Bruce AT et al (2005) Interferon-gamma and cancer immunoediting. Immunol Res 32:231-245. https://doi.org/10.1385/ir:32:1-3: 231
3. Ferris RL (2015) Immunology and immunotherapy of head and neck cancer. J Clin Oncol 33:3293-3304. https://doi.org/10.1200/JCO.2015.61.1509
4. Concha-Benavente F, Srivastava R, Ferrone S et al (2016) Immunological and clinical significance of HLA class I antigen processing machinery component defects in malignant cells. Oral Oncol 58:52-58. https://doi.org/10.1016/j.oraloncology.2016.05.008
5. Ferris RL, Hunt JL, Ferrone S (2005) Human leukocyte antigen (HLA) class I defects in head and neck cancer. Immunol Res 33:113-133. https://doi.org/10.1385/IR:33:2:113
6. Lee MY, Jeon JW, Sievers C et al (2020) Antigen processing and presentation in cancer immunotherapy. J Immunother Cancer. https://doi.org/10.1136/jitc-2020-001111
7. Leibowitz MS, Andrade Filho PA, Ferrone S et al (2011) Deficiency of activated STAT1 in head and neck cancer cells mediates TAP1-dependent escape from cytotoxic T lymphocytes. Cancer Immunol Immunother 60:525-535. https://doi.org/10.1007/s00262-010-0961-7
8. Leibowitz MS, Srivastava RM, Andrade Filho PA et al (2013) SHP2 is overexpressed and inhibits pSTAT1-mediated APM component expression, T-cell attracting chemokine secretion, and CTL recognition in head and neck cancer cells. Clin Cancer Res 19:798-808. https://doi.

org/10.1158/1078-0432.CCR-12-1517

9. Lopez-Albaitero A, Nayak JV, Ogino T et al (2006) Role of antigen-processing machinery in the in vitro resistance of squamous cell carcinoma of the head and neck cells to recognition by CTL. J Immunol 176:3402-3409. https://doi.org/10.4049/jimmunol.176.6.3402

10. Meissner M, Reichert TE, Kunkel M et al (2005) Defects in the human leukocyte antigen class I antigen processing machinery in head and neck squamous cell carcinoma: association with clinical outcome. Clin Cancer Res 11:2552-2560. https://doi.org/10.1158/1078-0432.CCR-04-2146

11. Yoshihama S, Roszik J, Downs I et al (2016) NLRC5/MHC class I transactivator is a target for immune evasion in cancer. Proc Natl Acad Sci U S A 113:5999-6004. https://doi.org/10.1073/pnas.1602069113

12. Zhu K, Wang J, Zhu J, Jiang J et al (1999) p53 induces TAP1 and enhances the transport of MHC class I peptides. Oncogene 18:7740-7747. https://doi.org/10.1038/sj.onc.1203235

13. Keck MK, Zuo Z, Khattri A et al (2015) Integrative analysis of head and neck cancer identifies two biologically distinct HPV and three non-HPV subtypes. Clin Cancer Res 21:870-881. https://doi.org/10.1158/1078-0432.CCR-14-2481

14. Tran L, Allen CT, Xiao R et al (2017) Cisplatin Alters antitumor immunity and synergizes with PD-1/PD-L1 inhibition in head and neck squamous cell carcinoma. Cancer Immunol Res 5(12):1141-1151. https://doi.org/10.1158/2326-6066.CIR-17-0235

15. Morisada M, Clavijo PE, Moore E et al (2018) PD-1 blockade reverses adaptive immune resistance induced by high-dose hypofractionated but not low-dose daily fractionated radiation. Onco Targets Ther. https://doi.org/10.1080/2162402X.2017.1395996

16. Baruah P, Lee M, Odutoye T et al (2012) Decreased levels of alternative co-stimulatory receptors OX40 and 4-1BB characterise T cells from head and neck cancer patients. Immunobiology 217:669-675. https://doi.org/10.1016/j.imbio.2011.11.005

17. Pfannenstiel LW, Diaz-Montero CM, Tian YF et al (2019) Immune-checkpoint blockade opposes CD8(+) T-cell suppression in human and murine cancer. Cancer Immunol Res 7:510-525. https://doi.org/10.1158/2326-6066.CIR-18-0054

18. Camacho M, Leon X, Fernandez-Figueras MT et al (2008) Prostaglandin E(2) pathway in head and neck squamous cell carcinoma. Head Neck 30:1175-1181. https://doi.org/10.1002/hed.20850

19. Dasgupta S, Bhattacharya-Chatterjee M, O'Malley BW et al (2005) Inhibition of NK cell activity through TGF-1 by down-regulation of NKG2D in a murine model of head and neck cancer. J Immunol 175:5541-5550. https://doi.org/10.4049/jimmunol.175.8.5541

20. Pak AS, Wright MA, Matthews JP et al (1995) Mechanisms of immune suppression in patients with head and neck cancer: presence of CD34(+) cells which suppress immune functions within cancers that secrete granulocyte-macrophage colony-stimulating factor. Clin Cancer Res 1(1):95-103

21. Davis RJ, Van Waes C, Allen CT (2016) Overcoming barriers to effective immunotherapy: MDSCs, TAMs, and Tregs as mediators of the immunosuppressive microenvironment in head and neck cancer. Oral Oncol 58:59-70. https://doi.org/10.1016/j.oraloncology.2016.05.002

22. Vasquez-Dunddel D, Pan F, Zeng Q et al (2013) STAT3 regulates arginase-I in myeloid-derived suppressor cells from cancer patients. J Clin Invest 123:1580-1589. https://doi.org/10.1172/JCI60083

23. Zhong LM, Liu ZG, Zhou X et al (2019) Expansion of PMN-myeloid derived suppressor cells

and their clinical relevance in patients with oral squamous cell carcinoma. Oral Oncol 95:157-163. https://doi.org/10.1016/j.oraloncology.2019.06.004
24. Lang S, Bruderek K, Kaspar C et al (2018) Clinical relevance and suppressive capacity of human myeloid-derived suppressor cell subsets. Clin Cancer Res 24:4834-4844. https://doi.org/10.1158/1078-0432.CCR-17-3726
25. Costa NL, Valadares MC, Souza PPC et al (2013) Tumor-associated macrophages and the profile of inflammatory cytokines in oral squamous cell carcinoma. Oral Oncol 49:216-223. https://doi.org/10.1016/j.oraloncology.2012.09.012
26. Cao X, Cai SF, Fehniger TA et al (2007) Granzyme B and perforin are important for regulatory T cell-mediated suppression of tumor clearance. Immunity 27:635-646. https://doi.org/10.1016/j.immuni.2007.08.014
27. Deaglio S, Dwyer KM, Gao W et al (2007) Adenosine generation catalyzed by CD39 and CD73 expressed on regulatory T cells mediates immune suppression. J Exp Med 204:1257-1265. https://doi.org/10.1084/jem.20062512
28. Badoual C, Hans S, Rodriguez J et al (2006) Prognostic value of tumor-infiltrating CD4+ T-cell subpopulations in head and neck cancers. Clin Cancer Res 12:465-472. https://doi.org/10.1158/1078-0432.CCR-05-1886
29. Qi Z, Liu Y, Mints M et al (2021) Single-cell deconvolution of head and neck squamous cell carcinoma. Cancers (Basel). https://doi.org/10.3390/cancers13061230
30. Strauss L, Bergmann C, Gooding W et al (2007) The frequency and suppressor function of CD4+CD25highFoxp3+ T cells in the circulation of patients with squamous cell carcinoma of the head and neck. Clin Cancer Res 13:6301-6311. https://doi.org/10.1158/1078-0432.CCR-07-1403
31. Frazer IH (2009) Interaction of human papillomaviruses with the host immune system: a well evolved relationship. Virology 384:410-414. https://doi.org/10.1016/j.virol.2008.10.004
32. Nasman A, Romanitan M, Nordfors C et al (2012) Tumor infiltrating CD8+ and Foxp3+ lymphocytes correlate to clinical outcome and human papillomavirus (HPV) status in tonsillar cancer. PLoS One. https://doi.org/10.1371/journal.pone.0038711
33. Stanley MA, Pett MR, Coleman N (2007) HPV: from infection to cancer. Biochem Soc Trans 35:1456-1460. https://doi.org/10.1042/BST0351456
34. Kanodia S, Fahey LM, Kast WM (2007) Mechanisms used by human papillomaviruses to escape the host immune response. Curr Cancer Drug Targets 7:79-89. https://doi.org/10.2174/156800907780006869
35. Bodily J, Laimins LA (2011) Persistence of human papillomavirus infection: keys to malignant progression. Trends Microbiol 19:33-39. https://doi.org/10.1016/j.tim.2010.10.002
36. O'Brien PM, Saveria Campo M (2002) Evasion of host immunity directed by papillomavirus-encoded proteins. Virus Res 88:103-117. https://doi.org/10.1016/s0168-1702(02)00123-5
37. Stanley M (2008) Immunobiology of HPV and HPV vaccines. Gynecol Oncol 109(Suppl. 2):S15-S21. https://doi.org/10.1016/j.ygyno.2008.02.003
38. Vu HL, Sikora AG, Fu S, Kao J (2010) HPV-induced oropharyngeal cancer, immune response and response to therapy. Cancer Lett 288:149-155. https://doi.org/10.1016/j.canlet.2009.06.026
39. Chang YE, Laimins LA (2000) Microarray analysis identifies interferon-inducible genes and Stat-1 as major transcriptional targets of human papillomavirus type 31. J Virol 74:4174-4182. https://doi.org/10.1128/jvi.74.9.4174-4182.2000
40. Nees M, Geoghegan JM, Hyman T et al (2001) Papillomavirus type 16 oncogenes downregulate

expression of interferon-responsive genes and upregulate proliferation-associated and NF-kappaB-responsive genes in cervical keratinocytes. J Virol 75:4283-4296. https://doi.org/10.1128/JVI.75.9.4283-4296.2001
41. Hayes DN, Van Waes C, Seiwert TY (2015) Genetic landscape of human papillomavirus-associated head and neck cancer and comparison to tobacco-related tumors. J Clin Oncol 33:3227-3234. https://doi.org/10.1200/JCO.2015.62.1086
42. Bhat P, Mattarollo SR, Gosmann C et al (2011) Regulation of immune responses to HPV infection and during HPV-directed immunotherapy. Immunol Rev 239:85-98. https://doi.org/10.1111/j.1600-065X.2010.00966.x
43. Zhou Q, Zhu K, Cheng H (2013) Toll-like receptors in human papillomavirus infection. Arch Immunol Ther Exp 61:203–215. https://doi.org/10.1007/s00005-013-0220-7
44. Albers A, Abe K, Hunt J et al (2005) Antitumor activity of human papillomavirus type 16 E7-specific T cells against virally infected squamous cell carcinoma of the head and neck. Cancer Res 65:11146-11155. https://doi.org/10.1158/0008-5472.CAN-05-0772
45. Gildener-Leapman N, Ferris RL, Bauman JE (2013) Promising systemic immunotherapies in head and neck squamous cell carcinoma. Oral Oncol 49:1089-1096. https://doi.org/10.1016/j.oraloncology.2013.09.009
46. Vambutas A, DeVoti J, Pinn W et al (2001) Interaction of human papillomavirus type 11 E7 protein with TAP-1 results in the reduction of ATP-dependent peptide transport. Clin Immunol 101:94-99. https://doi.org/10.1006/clim.2001.5094
47. Allen CT, Lewis JS Jr, El-Mofty SK et al (2010) Human papillomavirus and oropharynx cancer: biology, detection and clinical implications. Laryngoscope 120:1756-1772. https://doi.org/10.1002/lary.20936
48. Badoual C, Hans S, Merillon N et al (2013) PD-1-expressing tumor-infiltrating T cells are a favorable prognostic biomarker in HPV-associated head and neck cancer. Cancer Res 73:128-138. https://doi.org/10.1158/0008-5472.CAN-12-2606
49. Kansy BA, Concha-Benavente F, Srivastava RM et al (2017) PD-1 Status in CD8(+) T cells associates with survival and anti-PD-1 therapeutic outcomes in head and neck cancer. Cancer Res 77:6353-6364. https://doi.org/10.1158/0008-5472.CAN-16-3167

第 2 章 头颈部肿瘤免疫治疗临床开发中的药物靶点与策略

Drug Targets and Strategies in the Clinical Development of Immunotherapy for Head and Neck Cancer

（Athénaïs van der Elst，Jean-Pascal Machiels 著）

（茅芯慧，田素青 译）

摘要

复发和（或）转移性头颈部鳞状细胞癌（R/M HNSCC）是一种预后较差的恶性肿瘤，其治疗是肿瘤学领域的重大挑战。长期以来，对于铂类药物敏感的 R/M HNSCC 患者，EXTREME 方案 [顺铂或卡铂＋氟尿嘧啶（5-FU）＋西妥昔单抗] 一直被视为标准治疗方案。然而，对于铂类治疗失败的患者，二线治疗（如甲氨蝶呤、西妥昔单抗或紫杉醇类药物）的疗效有限，中位生存期通常不足 6 个月。得益于

原作者信息

A. van der Elst
Institute for Experimental and Clinical Research (IREC, pôle MIRO), Université catholique de Louvain (UCLouvain), Brussels, Belgium
e-mail: athenais.vanderelst@uclouvain.be

J.-P. Machiels (✉)
Institute for Experimental and Clinical Research (IREC, pôle MIRO), Université catholique de Louvain (UCLouvain), Brussels, Belgium

Department of Medical Oncology, Institut Roi Albert II, Cliniques universitaires Saint-Luc, Brussels, Belgium
e-mail: jean-pascal.machiels@uclouvain.be

CHECKMATE-141试验、KEYNOTE-012试验、KEYNOTE-055试验和KEYNOTE-040试验的研究成果，两种PD-1抑制剂——纳武利尤单抗和帕博利珠单抗——已被批准用于铂类治疗后进展的R/M HNSCC患者。此外，KEYNOTE-048试验的结果促使帕博利珠单抗进一步被批准作为R/M HNSCC患者的一线治疗方案，可作为单药治疗或与铂类及5-FU联合使用。目前，对于R/M HNSCC患者已有多种治疗方案可供选择，治疗决策主要基于PD-L1表达的联合阳性评分（CPS）、患者症状、对肿瘤快速缩小的需求、潜在的自身免疫性疾病以及化疗禁忌证。尽管PD-1抑制剂在部分患者中显示出卓越的长期疗效，但总缓解率仍有待提升。为进一步提高疗效，研究者们正在探索多种创新策略，包括免疫治疗间的联合应用，以及免疫治疗与靶向治疗、化疗或其他治疗模式的联合应用等。

关键词

抗CTLA-4 · 抗PD-1 · R/M HNSCC · 治疗指南

1　引言

头颈部鳞状细胞癌（HNSCC）起源于上皮细胞，常见于口腔、口咽、下咽和喉部。HNSCC是全球第七大常见恶性肿瘤，每年新发病例约70万例，2018年导致约35万人死亡[1]。

HNSCC的发生是多因素驱动的，其中吸烟和酒精摄入是主要危险因素，与75%~85%的HNSCC病例相关[2]。对于口咽癌而言，人乳头瘤病毒（HPV）感染是另一重要危险因素。HPV相关口咽癌的发病率正在增加，在全球范围内差异显著，HPV相关口咽癌估计约占口咽癌总数的30%[3]。HPV阳性的口咽癌患者预后显著优于HPV阴性患者，但发生在口咽以外部位的HPV阳性HNSCC较为罕见（<6%）[2]。

HNSCC的根治性治疗取决于原发肿瘤的部位及疾病分期。早期肿瘤[美国癌症联合委员会（American Joint Committee on Cancer, AJCC）Ⅰ期和Ⅱ期]通常采用单一治疗模式，如手术切除或根治性放疗。局部晚期疾病（AJCC Ⅲ期和Ⅳ期）患者则需接受多模式根治性治疗，包括化放疗或手术联合化放疗。尽管进行了积极的多模式治疗，超过50%的局部晚期HNSCC患者仍会出现远处转移和（或）局部或区域性复发。在某些特定情况下，局部或区域性复发的患者仍能从挽救性手术或再次放疗等治愈性治疗策略中获益[4]。

对于无法通过挽救性手术、放疗或两者联合治疗的局部复发性肿瘤患者，其预后与转移性疾病相似，未经治疗的中位生存期仅为6~9个月[4]。少数（<5%）患者在初诊时即表现为转移性疾病[2]。

直到最近，R/M HNSCC的一线姑息性全身治疗主要为铂类化疗联合西妥昔单抗（靶向表皮生长因子受体的单克隆抗体）[5]。2019年，帕博利珠单抗（一种靶向PD-1的单克隆抗体）被批准用于一线治疗R/M HNSCC患者，可以单药治疗或与化疗联合使用[6]。

PD-1是一种表达于活化T细胞表面的受体，与其配体PD-L1和PD-L2相互作用。在健康的免疫系统中，这种相互作用能够防止过度的炎症或自身免疫反应。然而，肿瘤细胞和（或）免疫细胞表达PD-L1会削弱T细胞效应活性，从而使肿瘤逃避免疫监视。通过抗PD-1或抗PD-L1药物阻断PD-1及其配体的相互作用，可以增强肿瘤内的免疫反应，进而可能导致肿瘤缩小[7]。目前，帕博利珠单抗和纳武利尤单抗是两种被批准用于治疗R/M HNSCC的免疫检查点抑制剂，均靶向PD-1[2]。

本章重点介绍与PD-1/PD-L1抑制剂相关的关键性研究，简述了确定治疗选择时需要考虑的主要因素，探讨了应用PD-1抑制剂时患者管理的核心内容，最后讨论了在R/M HNSCC中如何优化抗PD-1治疗。

2 抗PD-1治疗复发/转移性头颈部鳞状细胞癌

2.1 抗PD-1：从铂类治疗失败到一线治疗

2.1.1 在铂类治疗后使用纳武利尤单抗和帕博利珠单抗

帕博利珠单抗和纳武利尤单抗的疗效最初是在R/M HNSCC患

者中进行评估，这些患者在接受铂类治疗后病情进展。在Ⅰb期 KEYNOTE-012 试验中，帕博利珠单抗在 R/M HNSCC 患者中显示出持久的疗效，总缓解率（overall response rate, ORR）为 18%，并且很重要的一点是，其中 71% 的缓解持续时间超过 12 个月。中位总生存期（overall survival, OS）为 8 个月，1 年生存率为 38%（表 2-1）。治疗相关不良事件（treatment-related adverse event, TRAE）发生率为 64%，其中 3~4 级 TRAE 的发生率为 13%[8]。基于 KEYNOTE-012 试验中观察到的疗效和安全性，美国食品药品监督管理局（FDA）于 2016 年 8 月加速批准帕博利珠单抗用于铂类化疗后病情进展的 R/M HNSCC 患者（图 2-1）。Ⅱ期 KEYNOTE-055 试验和Ⅲ期 KEYNOTE-040 试验进一步验证了 KEYNOTE-012 试验的结果（表 2-1）[9]。

KEYNOTE-012 试验的结果在Ⅱ期 KEYNOTE-055 试验[9]和Ⅲ期 KEYNOTE-040 试验中得到了证实（表 2-1）。KEYNOTE-040 试验纳入了在铂类治疗期间或铂类治疗后 3~6 个月内疾病进展的 HNSCC 患者（患者接受的铂类治疗可能是针对 R/M 疾病或作为多模式根治性治疗的一部分）。患者按 1∶1 的比例随机分组接受帕博利珠单抗治疗或三种标准治疗（standard of care treatments, SOC）之一（即甲氨蝶呤、多西他赛或西妥昔单抗，由研究者决定）。试验结果显示，与研究者选择的标准治疗相比，帕博利珠单抗治疗组的中位 OS 有延长趋势（中位 OS 分别为 8.4 个月和 6.9 个月），但未达到统计学显著性：死亡风险比（hazard ratio, HR）为 0.80（95%CI：0.65~0.98；P=0.0161）。帕博利珠单抗组的 1 年生存率为 37%，而 SOC 组为 26.5%。尽管帕博利珠单抗组的缓解率中等（14.6% 对比 SOC 组的 10.1%），但帕博利珠单抗组的中位缓解持续时间显著优于 SOC 组（18.4 个月对比 5 个月）[10]。

纳武利尤单抗在二线治疗中也显示出显著的疗效。CHECKMATE-141 试验是一项随机、开放标签、Ⅲ期临床试验，比较了纳武利尤单抗与单药 SOC 治疗（甲氨蝶呤、多西他赛或西妥昔单抗）在 R/M HNSCC 患者中的疗效，这些患者在铂类治疗后 6 个月内出现疾病进展或复发（该试验为 2∶1 随机分组）。结果显示，纳武利尤单抗组的中位 OS 显著优于 SOC 组：7.5 个月对比 5.1 个月（HR=0.7，97.73%CI：0.51~0.96，P=0.01）（表 2-1）。无论 SOC 药物类型如何，纳武利尤单抗组的中

表 2-1 在铂类药物耐药的复发/转移性头颈部鳞状细胞癌患者中进行的抗 PD-1 研究[8-12]

研究	临床分期	药物名称	患者数	总缓解率(95% CI)	中位缓解持续时间/月（范围）	中位无进展生存期/月(95% CI)	中位总生存期/月(95% CI)	1年总生存率(95% CI)	2年总生存率(95% CI)	3级及以上治疗相关不良事件发生率
KEYNOTE-012[8]	Ib	帕博利珠单抗	192（汇总）	18% (13%~24%)	NR(2+~30+)		8 (6~10)	38%		13%
KEYNOTE-055[9]	II	帕博利珠单抗	171	16% (11%~23%)	8 (2+~12+)	2.1 (2.1~2.1)	8 (6~11)			15%
KEYNOTE-040[10]	III	帕博利珠单抗	247	14.6% (10.4%~19.6%)	18.4	2.1 (2.1~2.3)	8.4 (6.4~9.4)	37.0% (31.0~43.1)		13%
		IC	248	10.6% (6.6%~14.5%)	5.0	2.3 (2.1~2.8)	6.9 (5.9~8.0)	26.5% (21.2~32.2)		36%
CHECKMATE-141[11-12]	III	纳武利尤单抗	240	13.3% (2.1%~9.3%)	9.7	2.0 (1.9~2.1)	7.5 (5.5~9.1)	36% (28.5~43.4)	16.9% (12.4~22)	13%
		IC	121	5.8% (2.4%~11.6%)	4.0	2.3 (1.9~3.1)	5.1 (4.0~6.0)	16.6% (8.6~26.8)	6.0% (2.7~11.3)	35%
						HR=0.89 (0.7~1.13) P = 0.32	HR=0.80 (0.65~0.98) P = 0.0161			
							HR=0.70 (0.51~0.96) P = 0.01			

CI：置信区间；IC：研究者选择（西妥昔单抗、多西他赛、甲氨蝶呤）；HR：风险比；NR：未达到。

位 OS 均显著延长：甲氨蝶呤组中位 OS 为 4.6 个月（HR=0.64，95%CI：0.43~0.96）、多西他赛组中位 OS 为 5.8 个月（HR=0.82，95%CI：0.53~1.28）、西妥昔单抗组中位 OS 为 4.1 个月（HR=0.47，95%CI：0.22~1.01）。两组在无进展生存期（PFS）方面差异不显著（HR=0.89，95%CI：0.70~1.13，P=0.32）[11-12]。基于这些结果，FDA 于 2016 年 11 月批准纳武利尤单抗用于铂类治疗耐药的 HNSCC 患者，随后欧洲药品管理局（EMA）于 2017 年 3 月也批准了该适应证（图 2-1）。

以上两项将纳武利尤单抗和帕博利珠单抗与标准治疗方案比较的 Ⅲ 期临床试验的安全性结果倾向于支持抗 PD-1 治疗。在这两项试验中，抗 PD-1 治疗组患者中 3 级或 4 级治疗相关不良事件的发生率为 13%，而 SOC 组为 35%~36%[10-11]。有趣的是，上述试验还评估了生活质量（quality of life, QoL）。在 CHECKMATE-141 试验中，纳武利尤单抗稳定了患者的症状和功能，并延迟了患者报告的生活质量恶化的时间，而 SOC 组的细胞毒性化疗导致了生活质量的恶化[13]。同样，在 KEYNOTE-040 试验中，接受帕博利珠单抗治疗的患者的整体健康状态（global health status, GHS）和生活质量保持稳定，而 SOC 组在研究第 15 周时患者显示出 GHS 和 QoL 的轻度下降[14]。

2.1.2 帕博利珠单抗作为复发/转移性头颈部鳞状细胞癌的一线治疗

KEYNOTE-048 是一项三臂 Ⅲ 期研究，该试验进行了两种比较：①比较帕博利珠单抗单药治疗与铂类药物 +5-FU+ 西妥昔单抗（EXTREME 方案）；②比较帕博利珠单抗 + 铂类药物 +5-FU 与 EXTREME 方案。试验的共同主要终点为总生存期（OS）和无进展生存期（PFS）。结果根据 PD-L1 表达的联合阳性评分（combined positive score, CPS）和总人群进行分析：分为 CPS ≥ 1、CPS ≥ 20，以及总人群[6]。本试验的结果总结在表 2-2 和表 2-3 中。

在意向性治疗人群（intent-to-treat population, ITT）中，帕博利珠单抗单药治疗的中位 OS 为 11.5 个月，与 EXTREME 方案的 10.7 个月相比不具有劣势（表 2-2）。帕博利珠单抗组的总缓解率（ORR）为 16.9%，与铂类耐药患者的 ORR 相当，而 EXTREME 方案组为 36%。

第 2 章 头颈部肿瘤免疫治疗临床开发中的药物靶点与策略

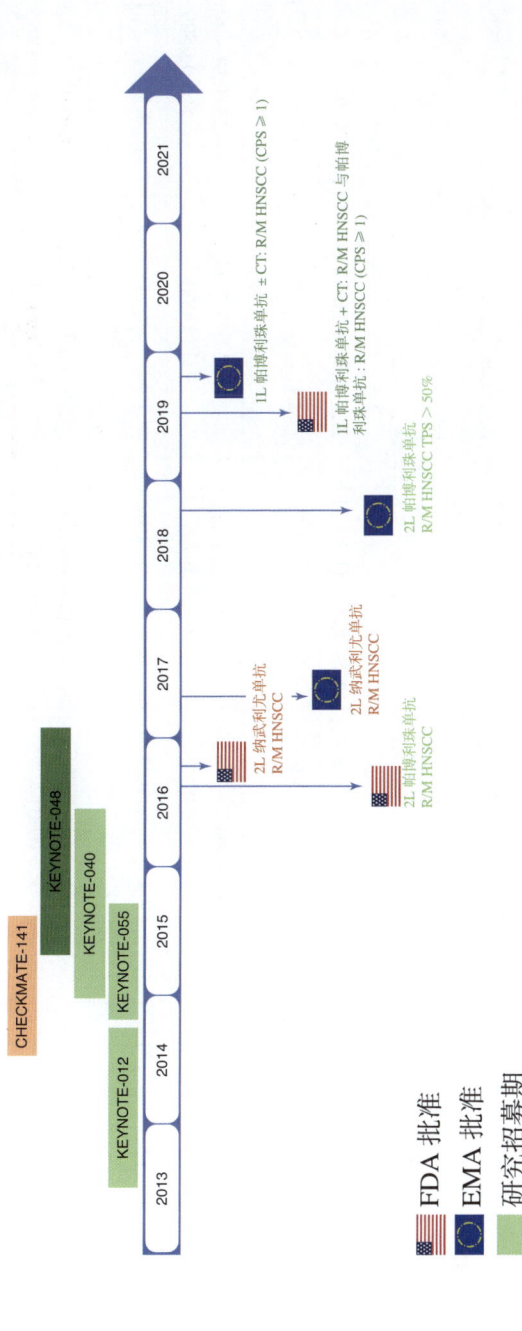

图 2-1 头颈部鳞状细胞癌（HNSCC）的免疫检查点抑制剂批准情况。2L：二线治疗；1L：一线治疗；R/M HNSCC：复发/转移性头颈部鳞状细胞癌；CT：化疗；TPS：肿瘤比例评分；CPS：联合阳性评分

表 2-2　KEYNOTE-048 试验：帕博利珠单抗单药治疗对比 EXTREME 方案[6,18]

药物名称	总意向性治疗人群 帕博利珠单抗	总意向性治疗人群 EXTREME	PD-L1 CPS≥1 帕博利珠单抗	PD-L1 CPS≥1 EXTREME	PD-L1 CPS≥20 帕博利珠单抗	PD-L1 CPS≥20 EXTREME	PD-L1 CPS<1 帕博利珠单抗	PD-L1 CPS<1 EXTREME	1≤PD-L1 CPS<20 帕博利珠单抗	1≤PD-L1 CPS<20 EXTREME
患者数	301	300	257	255	133	122	44	45	124	133
总缓解率	17%	36%	19%	35%	23%	36%	4%	42%	14%	34%
完全缓解率	5%	3%	5%	3%	8%	3%				
部分缓解率	12%	33%	14%	32%	16%	33%				
疾病稳定率	27%	34%	28%	33%	30%	35%				
疾病进展率	40%	12%	39%	13%	32%	10%				
中位缓解持续时间/月（范围）	22.6 (1.5~43)	4.5 (1.2~38.7+)	23.4 (1.5~43+)	4.5 (1.2~38.7+)	22.6 (2.7~43+)	4.2 (1.2~31.5)	2.6 (2.2~3.0)	7.8 (2.0~38.6+)	NR (1.5~38.9+)	5.0 (1.4~38.7+)
中位无进展生存期/月	2.3	5.2	3.2	5.0	3.4	5.3	2.1	6.2	2.2	4.9
HR (95% CI), P 值	1.29 (1.09~1.53), P=0.9983		1.13 (0.94~1.36), P=0.8958		0.99 (0.76~1.29), P=0.4679		4.31 (2.63~7.08), P=1.0000		1.25 (0.96~1.61), P=0.9509	
中位总生存期/月	11.5	10.7	12.3	10.3	14.8	10.7	7.9	11.3	10.8	10.1
HR (95% CI), P 值	0.83 (0.70~0.99), P=0.0198		0.74 (0.61~0.90), P=0.0013		0.58 (0.44~0.78), P=0.0001		1.51 (0.96~2.37), P=0.9624		0.86 (0.66~1.12), P=0.1283	
1 年总生存率	49%	44%	50%	44%	56%	45%	39%	49%	44%	42%
2 年总生存率	27%	19%	29%	17%	35%	19%	16%	27%	22%	16%
3 级及以上治疗相关不良事件发生率	17%	69%								

CPS：联合阳性评分；EXTREME：铂类药物 -5-FU - 西妥昔单抗方案；CI：置信区间；HR：风险比。

表 2-3 KEYNOTE-048 试验：帕博利珠单抗联合化疗对比 EXTREME 方案 [6, 18]

药物名称	总意向性治疗人群		PD-L1 CPS≥1		PD-L1 CPS≥20		PD-L1 CPS<1		1≤PD-L1 CPS<20	
	帕博利珠单抗+化疗	EXTREME	帕博利珠单抗+化疗	EXTREME	帕博利珠单抗+化疗	EXTREME	帕博利珠单抗+化疗	EXTREME	帕博利珠单抗+化疗	EXTREME
患者数	281	278	242	235	126	110	39	43	116	125
总缓解率（ORR）	36%	36%	36%	36%	43%	38%	31%	40%	29%	34%
完全缓解率	6%	3%	7%	3%	10%	4%				
部分缓解率	30%	33%	30%	33%	33%	35%				
疾病稳定率	28%	34%	26%	33%	23%	35%				
疾病进展率	17%	12%	17%	12%	15%	8%				
中位缓解持续时间/月（范围）	6.7 (1.7~39.1)	4.3 (1.2~31.5+)	6.7 (1.6~39.0+)	4.5 (1.2~38.7+)	7.1 (2.1~39.0+)	4.2 (1.2~31.5+)	5.7 (2.6~20.6+)	4.3 (2.0~31.2+)	5.6 (1.6~25.6+)	5.0 (1.4~38.7+)
中位无进展生存期/月	4.9	5.1	5.1	5.0	5.8	5.3	4.7	6.2	4.9	4.9
HR (95% CI), P 值	0.93 (0.78~1.11), $P=0.212$		0.84 (0.69~1.02), $P=0.037$		0.76 (0.58~1.01), $P=0.030$		1.46 (0.93~2.3), $P=0.94989$		0.93 (0.71~1.21), $P=0.29189$	

（续表）

药物名称	总意向性治疗人群		PD-L1 CPS≥1		PD-L1 CPS≥20		PD-L1 CPS<1		1≤PD-L1 CPS<20	
	帕博利珠单抗+化疗	EXTREME	帕博利珠单抗+化疗	EXTREME	帕博利珠单抗+化疗	EXTREME	帕博利珠单抗+化疗	EXTREME	帕博利珠单抗+化疗	EXTREME
中位总生存期/月	13.0	10.7	13.6	10.4	14.7	11	11.3	10.7	12.7	9.9
HR (95% CI), P值	0.72 (0.60~0.87), P=0.00025		0.65 (0.53~0.80), P=0.000002		0.60 (0.45~0.82), P=0.00044		1.21 (0.076~1.94), P=0.78932		0.71 (0.54~0.94), P=0.00726	
1年总生存率	53%	44%	55%	44%	57%	46%	41%	46%	53%	41%
2年总生存率	29%	18%	31%	17%	35%	19%	20%	26%	26%	14%
3级及以上治疗相关不良事件发生率	72%	69%								

CPS：联合阳性评分；EXTREME：铂类药物-5-FU-西妥昔单抗方案；CI：置信区间；HR：风险比。

然而，帕博利珠单抗组的中位 PFS 低于 EXTREME 方案组（分别为 2.3 个月和 5.2 个月）。值得注意的是，帕博利珠单抗组的缓解持续时间显著更长，达到 22.6 个月，而 EXTREME 方案组仅为 4.5 个月。此外，生存曲线在前 7~8 个月中倾向于 EXTREME 方案，但在 8 个月后转而更有利于帕博利珠单抗单药治疗[6]。

在帕博利珠单抗中加入铂类药物和 5-FU 显著提高了总人群的 OS，中位 OS 为 13 个月，而 EXTREME 方案组为 10.7 个月。帕博利珠单抗联合化疗组的 ORR 为 35.6%，但中位缓解持续时间仅为 6.7 个月[6]（表 2-3）。有趣的是，与 EXTREME 方案相比，帕博利珠单抗单药治疗在生存曲线初期（早期死亡）显示的明显劣势在帕博利珠单抗联合化疗组中未被观察到[6]。

基于 KEYNOTE-048 试验的研究结果，美国 FDA 于 2019 年 6 月批准帕博利珠单抗单药治疗用于 PD-L1 阳性（CPS ≥ 1）的转移性或无法切除的复发性 HNSCC 患者的一线治疗，并批准其与铂类药物和 5-FU 联合使用（无论 CPS 状态）。2019 年 10 月，EMA 也批准了这一适应证，但帕博利珠单抗单药及其与铂类药物和 5-FU 的联合治疗均要求 CPS ≥ 1（图 2-1）[6]。

2.2 治疗选择

在复发 / 转移性头颈部鳞状细胞癌（R/M HNSCC）的一线治疗中批准的方案包括：①帕博利珠单抗单药治疗；②帕博利珠单抗加 5-FU 和卡铂 / 顺铂；③西妥昔单抗加 5-FU 和卡铂 / 顺铂（EXTREME 方案）。将顺铂 / 多西他赛和西妥昔单抗结合的 TPeX 是 EXTREME 方案的一种替代方案[2, 15]。为了为每个患者选择合适的治疗方案，临床医生应牢记治疗目标：症状控制、保持或改善生活质量、延长生存期[16]。这些目标可能会根据患者的愿望有所不同。因此，治疗选择应基于肿瘤特性（PD-L1 表达、肿瘤负荷、对铂类药物的敏感性和复发部位）和患者特性（表现状态、器官功能、并发症、症状和患者偏好）[17]。

2.2.1 PD-L1 表达

在上述试验中，PD-L1 表达被作为预测治疗效果的生物标志物进行评估。PD-L1 表达可以通过联合阳性评分（combined positive score, CPS）或肿瘤比例评分（tumor proportion score, TPS）来测量。CPS 的定义为 PD-L1 染色的肿瘤细胞和周围淋巴细胞及巨噬细胞的总和，除以所有存活肿瘤细胞的总数，再乘以 100。而 TPS 仅表示表达 PD-L1 的存活肿瘤细胞的比例[2]。

在 KEYNOTE-048 试验中，结果按 CPS 进行分层分析：CPS ≥ 1，CPS ≥ 20，以及总人群（表 2-2 和表 2-3）。对于 CPS < 1 及 CPS ≥ 1 到 CPS < 20 的亚组患者，因这些参数的统计分析并非预先设定，相关数据应谨慎解释[6, 18]。

在 CPS ≥ 20 的患者中，帕博利珠单抗组的中位总生存期（OS）显著优于 EXTREME 方案组，分别为 14.8 个月和 10.7 个月（表 2-2）。2 年生存率帕博利珠单抗组为 35.3%，而 EXTREME 方案组为 19.1%。总缓解率（ORR）帕博利珠单抗组为 23.5%，EXTREME 方案组为 36.1%；但帕博利珠单抗组的中位缓解持续时间更长，为 22.6 个月。在 CPS ≥ 20 的患者中，帕博利珠单抗联合铂类药物和 5-FU 相比 EXTREME 方案进一步提高了中位 OS，分别为 14.7 个月和 11.0 个月。联合治疗组的 ORR 为 43%，而 EXTREME 方案组为 38%。在无进展生存期（PFS）方面，帕博利珠单抗联合化疗组为 5.8 个月，而 EXTREME 方案组为 5.3 个月（表 2-3）[6, 10]。

在 CPS ≥ 1 的患者中，帕博利珠单抗组的中位 OS 显著延长，为 12.3 个月，而 EXTREME 方案组为 10.3 个月。然而，这一阳性结果很大程度上归因于 CPS ≥ 20 的患者，该亚组也包含在 CPS ≥ 1 人群中。事实上，在 CPS 为 1~19 的患者中，中位 OS 无显著差异：帕博利珠单抗组为 10.8 个月，EXTREME 方案组为 10.1 个月（HR=0.85，95%CI：0.66~1.12，P=0.1282）（表 2-2）[18]。

在 CPS < 1 的患者中，帕博利珠单抗单药治疗的疗效较弱，帕博利珠单抗组的 ORR 仅为 4.5%，而 EXTREME 方案组为 42.2%；中位 OS 分别为 7.9 个月和 11.3 个月（表 2-2）[18]。

KEYNOTE-048 试验的结果支持 CPS 对于预测帕博利珠单抗疗效有价值。因此，FDA 和 EMA 均以 CPS ≥ 1 作为批准帕博利珠单抗单药治疗用于一线治疗的依据。然而，值得注意的是，部分 CPS ≥ 20 的患者对 PD-1 抑制剂无反应，而部分 PD-L1 表达阴性的患者仍能从 PD-1 抑制剂治疗中获益[19]。因此，CPS 虽具有预测价值，但作为与此治疗反应的生物标志物不够完美，其机制也尚未被完全阐明。

2.2.2 症状和肿瘤负荷

在 KEYNOTE-048 试验中，即使在 CPS ≥ 20 的患者中，化疗联合西妥昔单抗（EXTREME 方案）在治疗前 8 个月内的生存率仍然高于帕博利珠单抗单药治疗。这表明，对于部分患者而言，帕博利珠单抗单药治疗可能导致较差的预后。这可能与帕博利珠单抗单药治疗的较低的缓解率（ORR）和较短的无进展生存期（PFS）有关（表 2-2）[6]。

对于肿瘤负荷较重的患者，若治疗反应迟缓或疾病迅速进展，则可能需要通过快速缩小肿瘤体积来避免早期死亡。此外，有研究表明，抗 PD-1 治疗在部分患者中可能需要数月才能诱导肿瘤缓解。在多数临床试验中，只要患者未出现显著的临床恶化，通常允许在疾病进展后继续治疗。尽管在 HNSCC 中，晚期肿瘤缓解的发生率尚未得到全面研究，但在 CHECKMATE-141 试验中，患者在出现 RECIST v1.1 标准定义的疾病进展后继续接受纳武利尤单抗治疗，25% 的患者（60 例中的 15 例）显示出一定程度的肿瘤缩小[20]。复发性/转移性 HNSCC 患者通常伴有严重的症状，包括疼痛、疲劳、吞咽困难、呼吸急促以及声音改变，这些症状显著影响患者的生活质量。此外，这些患者还面临较高的感染风险，并可能发生出血、气道阻塞、高钙血症或脊髓压迫等并发症[17]。在 SOCCER 试验中，Hecht 等 2020 年发现治疗效果与肿瘤相关症状的缓解有明确关联[16]。因此，对于症状严重（如疼痛和吞咽困难）、肿瘤负荷较重或存在出血及气道阻塞风险的患者，应优先选择具有较高缓解率的治疗方案，例如化疗联合帕博利珠单抗或化疗联合西妥昔单抗。在这些临床情境下，与单一免疫治疗相比，化疗通过快速缩小肿瘤体积可能在症状控制方面更加有效[2, 16]。

2.2.3 HPV 状态

HPV 引发的口咽癌（oropharyngeal cancer, OPC）与 HPV 阴性的头颈部鳞状细胞癌有不同的免疫微环境：它们具有更高的免疫细胞浸润和高度活跃的 CD8+ T 细胞[21]。然而，在不同的临床试验中，HPV 阳性的 OPC 并未显示出抗 PD-1 治疗的明显优势。在 KEYNOTE-012 研究中，HPV 相关疾病的总缓解率（ORR）更高（24% 对比 16%）[8]。在 KEYNOTE-055 研究中，HPV 阳性和阴性亚组的缓解率和生存率相似[9]。在 KEYNOTE-040 研究中，与 HPV 阳性 OPC 相比（HR=0.97，95%CI：0.63~1.49），HPV 阴性癌症似乎从帕博利珠单抗治疗中获益更多（HR=0.77，95%CI：0.6~0.97），但差异不显著[10]。相比之下，在 CHECKMATE-141 研究中，与接受纳武利尤单抗治疗的 HPV 阴性患者相比（HR=0.73，95%CI：0.42~1.25），接受纳武利尤单抗治疗的 HPV 阳性癌症患者更有可能获益（HR=0.56，95%CI：0.32~0.99）[11]。在 KEYNOTE-048 研究中，与 EXTREME 方案相比，帕博利珠单抗加化疗在 HPV 阳性 OPC 中的益处更为显著（HR=0.56，95%CI：0.36~0.87）[6]。

总的来说，无论是 HPV 阳性还是 HPV 阴性的头颈部鳞状细胞癌患者，都能从抗 PD-1 治疗中获益。因此，HPV 状态不应成为临床实践中选择治疗方案的决定性因素[22]。然而，这种情况未来可能会随着针对不同免疫检查点抑制剂的组合疗法的出现而改变[21]。

2.2.4 老年患者和体能状态差的患者

在头颈部鳞状细胞癌中，有较高比例的患者年龄在 65 岁以上。年龄可能对免疫系统功能及肿瘤微环境产生影响[23]。因此，明确年龄是否影响抗 PD-1 治疗的疗效具有重要意义。虽然老年患者并未被系统性地排除在前瞻性临床试验之外，但在大多数试验中老年患者属于代表性不足的群体。

在 CHECKMATE-141 试验的事后分析中，对 R/M HNSCC 铂类耐药患者按年龄分组（＜65 岁和≥65 岁）评估了纳武利尤单抗的疗效和安全性。结果显示，与研究者选择的治疗方案（SOC）相比，在两组中应用纳武利尤单抗均能获得更高的中位总生存期、更高的 12 个月生存率和更高的总缓解率。此外，纳武利尤单抗的耐受性良好，两组患者的治疗相关不良事件发生率和严重程度相当。进一步以70岁为年龄分界的分析显示，纳武利尤单抗在70岁及以上患者中的疗效和安全性与SOC类似，但由于样本量较少，该分析结果需要谨慎解读[23]。在KEYNOTE-048试验的亚组分析中，无论是年龄低于65岁还是高于65岁，帕博利珠单抗单药治疗在总人群、CPS≥1人群以及CPS≥20人群中，相较于西妥昔单抗联合化疗均表现出更优的风险比（HR）。帕博利珠单抗联合化疗的结果也支持这一趋势[6]。

基于上述这些研究结果，年龄不应成为选择抗PD-1治疗的限制性因素。

相比之下，体能状态差的患者（如ECOG评分≥2）是一个更具挑战性的群体。通常，ECOG评分≥2被视为细胞毒性化疗的相对禁忌证，但对抗PD-1单药治疗则不然。然而，由于此类患者通常被排除在前瞻性临床试验之外，目前尚不清楚PD-1抑制剂在这类患者中的疗效和安全性。鉴于抗PD-1单药治疗具有良好的毒性特征，并可能带来长期获益，可考虑为部分体能状态较差的患者提供此治疗。但由于免疫检查点抑制剂（immune checkpoint inhibitor, ICI）治疗费用较高，需要在肿瘤多学科团队中充分讨论后决定[24]。目前正在进行的开放标签、Ⅱ期随机前瞻性ELDORANDO试验（NCT03193931）纳入了ECOG评分为2的患者，该试验比较帕博利珠单抗与甲氨蝶呤作为R/M HNSCC老年患者、体能较弱患者或有顺铂禁忌证患者一线治疗的疗效和安全性，主要研究终点为OS。另一项包括ECOG评分为2患者的试验是TOPNIVO研究（NCT03226756）。这两项试验的结果将有助于阐明PD-1抑制剂在体能状态较差患者中的疗效和安全性，为这类患者的治疗决策提供重要依据。

3　患者使用免疫检查点抑制剂的管理

患者对免疫治疗的反应动力学与传统细胞毒性化疗显著不同，因此需要调整监测和管理策略。在使用ICI治疗时，可观察到一些独特且不常见的反应模式，如长期治疗获益、同一患者不同肿瘤部位之间的不一致反应、假性进展以及超进展[22]。本节将讨论假性进展和超进展，以及头颈部肿瘤患者特有的不良反应管理。

3.1 超进展

在接受免疫治疗后，部分患者会出现比预期更快的肿瘤生长，这种现象被称为超进展（hyperprogression）。关于超进展的定义存在多种标准。美国癌症免疫治疗学会（The Society for Immunotherapy of Cancer, SITC）定义：肿瘤生长速率（tumor growth rate,TGR）较预期速率至少增加2倍；其他定义：按照实体瘤反应评估标准（Response Evaluation Criteria in Solid Tumor, RECIST）初次评估时表现为疾病进展，并且参考期与试验期之间的TGR增加≥2倍；或肿瘤生长动力学比值（TGK比值）≥2[22]。

在接受ICI治疗的不同类型肿瘤中，超进展性疾病（hyperprogressive disease, HPD）的发生率约为4%～29%。针对头颈部肿瘤的首个回顾性研究分析了34例患者，其中29%的患者被诊断为HPD。该研究发现HPD与区域复发明显相关，并且与较短的无进展生存期（PFS）相关，但对OS的影响不显著[25]。更近期的回顾性研究涵盖了更多的患者（患者数量分别为120例、125例和49例），结果显示，HPD的发生率分别为18%、14.4%和15.4%，且HPD与较差的PFS和OS相关[26-28]。尽管如此，超进展的概念仍存在争议。目前尚不清楚观察到的加速肿瘤生长是由ICI治疗引发的，还是由于疾病本身的自然进程导致的。接受ICI治疗的HNSCC患者通常既往接受的治疗较多，可能已经处于快速肿瘤生长和临床恶化的高风险状态。对于伴随临床恶化的快速肿瘤生长的患者，应暂停治疗，并重新评估治疗策略。

3.2 假性进展和疾病进展后的持续治疗

假性进展（pseudoprogression）被定义为影像学显示的病灶直径初期增加，随后出现肿瘤缩小。生物学机制可能包括两种情况：①在抗肿瘤免疫反应充分启动之前，肿瘤继续生长；②免疫细胞浸润导致影像上肿瘤体积看似增加[29]。因此，传统的疗效评价标准（如RECIST v1.1）可能低估 ICI 的治疗获益[22]。大多数评估 ICI 的临床试验允许在患者出现 RECIST 标准定义的疾病进展后继续治疗，只要患者符合特定条件。在 CHECKMATE-141 试验中，如果患者的体能状态稳定，未出现快速疾病进展，并能耐受纳武利尤单抗的治疗，则可以在 RECIST v1.1 定义的疾病进展后继续治疗。在 240 例随机分配至纳武利尤单抗组的患者中，146 例符合 RECIST 定义的疾病进展，62 例继续接受治疗，其中 60 例可评估疗效。15 例（25%）的肿瘤负荷未发生变化，另有 15 例（25%）的靶病灶体积出现减少，其中 3 例（5%）的靶病灶缩小超过 30%。疾病进展后继续接受纳武利尤单抗治疗的患者中位 OS 为 12.7 个月，而总意向性治疗人群的中位 OS 为 7.7 个月[20]。这些结果表明，对于经过严格筛选的、临床稳定且未出现严重免疫相关毒性的患者，在疾病进展后继续接受 ICI 治疗可能带来一定的获益。

免疫特异性疗效评价标准已经被开发用于临床试验中的免疫治疗疗效评估，如免疫相关反应标准（immune-related response criteria, irRC）和免疫相关实体瘤反应评估标准（immune-related Response Evaluation Criteria in Solid Tumors, irRECIST）。上述两个标准均要求在初次出现疾病进展迹象后进行确认[22]。然而，这些免疫相关标准尚未涵盖所有免疫治疗中不典型的应答模式，且在日常临床实践中应用难度较大。因此，RECIST v1.1 仍应作为患者管理的标准评价工具[29]。

3.3 头颈部肿瘤患者的特异性毒性反应

免疫检查点抑制剂具有特定模式的毒性反应，这些毒性反应被称为免疫相关不良事件（immune-related adverse event, irAE），可累及任何器官系统[30]。临床试验表明，帕博利珠单抗和纳武利尤单抗的毒性特征相似，总体毒性水平低于标准化疗。在 CHECKMATE-141 试验和 KEYNOTE-040 试验中，接受抗 PD-1 治疗的患者中有 13% 发生了 3 级或 4 级治疗相关不良事件（TRAE），而研究者选择的治疗方案组该发生率分别为 37% 和 36%[10-11]。在 CHECKMATE-141 试验中，大部分 3~4 级不良事件发生在纳武利尤单抗治疗的前 6 个月内[12]。在 KEYNOTE-048 试验中，治疗相关的 3 级及以上不良事件的发生率为：帕博利珠单抗单药治疗组 17%，帕博利珠单抗联合化疗组 72%，西妥昔单抗联合化疗组 69%。最常见的免疫相关不良事件包括甲状腺功能减退和甲状腺功能亢进、肺炎、严重皮肤反应、输液反应、结肠炎、肝炎和肾炎[6]。对于头颈部肿瘤患者，irAE 管理的总体原则与其他实体瘤类似[22]，但需格外关注某些头颈部鳞状细胞癌患者可能有急性并发症的高风险，例如感染、气道阻塞和出血。在 KEYNOTE-048 试验中，肿瘤部位出血的风险在帕博利珠单抗单药治疗组和帕博利珠单抗联合化疗组中未显著增加，发生率分别为 7% 和 9%，而西妥昔单抗联合化疗组为 5%[6]。对于存在巨大肿瘤、气道阻塞风险或潜在出血并发症的患者，帕博利珠单抗联合化疗可能是更优选择。联合治疗方案能够更快速地缩小肿瘤体积，从而降低因免疫治疗引发的肿瘤炎症导致的急性气道阻塞风险。因此，在规划免疫治疗时，对气道阻塞的有效管理至关重要[17]。

4 优化抗 PD-1 治疗在复发/转移性头颈部鳞状细胞癌中的应用

尽管纳武利尤单抗和帕博利珠单抗这两种抗 PD-1 的单克隆抗体（monoclonal antibody，mAb）已经被证明可以改善患者生存率，但仍有多种治疗策略正在探索中，包括开发抗 PD-L1 药物，联合应用不同免疫检查点抑制剂，以及抗 PD-1/PD-L1 药物与靶向治疗或其他治疗模式联合应用。本节重点讨论关于抗 PD-1/PD-L1 药物单独应用或与抗 CTLA-4 联合应用的研究。

4.1 其他抗 PD-1/PD-L1 药物（单独应用或与抗 CTLA-4 药物联合应用）

除了纳武利尤单抗和帕博利珠单抗外，其他抗 PD-1/PD-L1 药物（PD-1/PD-L1 抑制剂）也正在 HNSCC 治疗中进行开发。其中一些药物已经被批准用于治疗其他类型的肿瘤，如阿替利珠单抗（atezolizumab）、阿维鲁单抗（avelumab）、西米普利单抗（cemiplimab）和度伐利尤单抗（durvalumab）[7]。

度伐利尤单抗是一种靶向 PD-L1 的单克隆抗体，已在多项临床试验中作为单药或与抗 CTLA-4 药物（如替西木单抗）联合治疗 HNSCC 患者，但尚未被批准用于 HNSCC。

CTLA-4 是一种表达于 T 细胞上的免疫检查点受体，通过调节淋巴结和组织中的 T 细胞活性发挥免疫抑制作用。阻断 CTLA-4 可以增强效应性 CD4+ T 细胞的功能，并抑制调节性 T 细胞对树突细胞的抑制功能，从而增强抗肿瘤免疫力。由于 PD-1 和 CTLA-4 具有不同的作用机制，联合阻断这两种免疫检查点可能对抗肿瘤免疫反应产生协同效应，从而提高疗效。这种联合疗法在转移性黑色素瘤中已显示出提高缓解率和延长生存期的潜力[7]。在 R/M HNSCC 中，抗 PD-1/PD-L1 药物和抗 CTLA-4 药物联合应用已在多个临床试验中进行了研究，但似乎未能改善 OS。

在铂类耐药患者中评估度伐利尤单抗单独应用或与替西木单抗（即 tremelimumab，是一种靶向 CTLA-4 的 mAb）联合应用的Ⅱ期和Ⅲ期临床试验的结果总结在表 2-4 中。

HAWK 试验是一项Ⅱ期单臂临床试验，该试验在 PD-L1 高表达（TPS ≥ 25%）的铂类耐药的 R/M HNSCC 患者中对作为二线治疗的度伐利尤单抗进行了评估。结果显示总缓解率（ORR）为 16.2%，中位无进展生存期（PFS）为 2.1 个月，中位总生存期（OS）为 7.1 个月（表 2-4）。该试验显示度伐利尤单抗毒性非常低，因为只有 8% 的患者出现了 3 级及以上的治疗相关不良事件[31]。

CONDOR 试验是另一项Ⅱ期临床试验，该试验招募了 PD-L1 低表达或阴性（TPS＜25%）的铂类耐药的 R/M HNSCC 患者。患者被随机分入度伐利尤单抗加替西木单抗的联合治疗组、度伐利尤单抗单药治疗组或替西木单抗单药治疗组。在度伐利尤单抗单药治疗组中，PFS 为 1.9 个月，中位 OS 为 6 个月。ORR 低于 HAWK 研究的 9.2%，可能是因为患者群体中 PD-L1 表达水平较低。替西木单抗单药治疗的活性很差，ORR 仅为 1.6%。在替西木单抗加度伐利尤单抗的联合治疗组中，ORR 为 7.8%，低于单用度伐利尤单抗的 9.2%[32]。

度伐利尤单抗单药治疗在Ⅲ期 EAGLE 试验中进一步被评估。在该试验中，铂类化疗后进展的患者被随机分配到度伐利尤单抗单药治疗组、度伐利尤单抗加替西木单抗的联合治疗组，以及标准治疗组（西妥

表 2-4 头颈部鳞状细胞癌的抗 PD-L1 和抗 CTLA-4 联合治疗[31-33]

研究	临床分期	药物名称	患者数	总缓解率(95%CI)	中位缓解持续时间/月(范围)	中位无进展生存期/月(95%CI)	中位总生存期/月(95%CI)	1年总生存率(95%CI)	2年总生存率(95%CI)	3级及以上治疗相关不良事件发生率
HAWK[31]	Ⅱ	度伐利尤单抗	111	16%(9.9%~24.4%)	10.3	2.1(1.9~3.7)	7.1(4.9~9.9)	33.6%		8%
CONDOR[32]	Ⅱ	度伐利尤单抗	67	9.2%(3.5%~19.0%)	NR	1.9(1.8~2.8)	6.0(4.0~11.3)	36%		12.3%
		替西木单抗	67	1.6%(0%~8.5%)	NR	1.9(1.8~2.0)	5.5(3.9~7.0)	24%		16.9%
		度伐利尤单抗+替西木单抗	133	7.8%(3.8%~13.8%)	9.4(4.9~NA)	2.0(1.9~2.1)	7.6(4.9~10.6)	37%		15.8%
EAGLE[33]	Ⅲ	度伐利尤单抗	240	17.9(13.3%~23.4%)	12.9(6.9~21.0)	2.1(1.9~3.0)	7.6(6.1~9.8)	37%	18.4%	10.1%
		度伐利尤单抗+替西木单抗	247	18.2(13.6%~23.6%)	7.4(3.6~14.8)	2.0(1.9~2.3)	6.5(5.5~8.2)	30.4%	13.3%	16.3%
		IC	249	17.3(12.8%~22.6%)	3.7(2.0~4.2)	3.7(3.1~3.7)	8.3(7.3~9.2)	30.5%	10.3%	24.2%
							度伐利尤单抗对比IC：HR=0.88(0.72~1.08)，$P=0.20$；度伐利尤单抗+替西木单抗对比IC：HR=1.04(0.85~1.26)，$P=0.76$			

CI：置信区间；IC：研究者选择（西妥昔单抗、紫杉烷类药物、甲氨蝶呤或氟嘧啶类药物）；HR：风险比；NR：未达到；NA：不适用。

昔单抗、紫杉烷类、甲氨蝶呤或氟嘧啶类）。该试验未达到主要终点，因为与标准治疗相比，无论是否加用替西木单抗，度伐利尤单抗都未能显著提高生存率[33]。然而，度伐利尤单抗单药治疗组的 ORR 为 17.9%，中位 PFS 为 12.9 个月，显示出度伐利尤单抗在这一人群中的临床活性。此外，该组中位 OS 为 7.6 个月，1 年生存率为 7%，与 KEYNOTE-040 研究和 CHECKMATE-141 研究中的帕博利珠单抗和纳武利尤单抗的结果相当[10-11, 33]。度伐利尤单抗加替西木单抗组的 ORR 为 18%，与度伐利尤单抗单药治疗相似。与单药治疗相比，联合治疗组的毒性更高（3 级及以上治疗相关不良事件发生率：16% 对比 10%）[33]。

尽管在铂类耐药患者中抗 PD-1/PD-L1 药物与抗 CTLA-4 药物联合应用未能显著提高生存期，但这一组合在 R/M HNSCC 的一线治疗中继续进行评估（CHECKMATE-741 试验、CHECKMATE-651 试验和 KESTREL 试验）。CHECKMATE-741 试验是一项双盲的 Ⅱ 期试验，比较了纳武利尤单抗加伊匹木单抗（即 ipilimumab，是一种抗 CTLA-4 药物）与纳武利尤单抗加安慰剂。总缓解率和缓解持续时间是主要终点[34]。最终结果尚待公布，但 2019 年 4 月的新闻稿宣布未达到主要终点[35]。CHECKMATE-651 试验是一项 Ⅲ 期试验，比较纳武利尤单抗加伊匹木单抗与 EXTREME 方案，主要终点是所有参与者和 PD-L1 高表达（CPS ≥ 20）的肿瘤患者的总生存期。主要终点未达成，然而，在 PD-L1 高表达（CPS ≥ 20）的肿瘤患者中观察到纳武利尤单抗加伊匹木单抗的正向总生存期趋势：17.6 个月对比 14.6 个月（HR=0.78, 95% CI：0.59~1.03）[36]。Ⅲ 期的 KESTREL 研究将度伐利尤单抗单药治疗或联合替西木单抗与 EXTREME 方案进行了比较。2021 年 2 月的新闻稿宣布，对于 PD-L1 高表达（TPS ≥ 50% 或 ≥ 25% 的肿瘤浸润性免疫细胞表达 PD-L1）的患者，与 EXTREME 方案相比，度伐利尤单抗单药治疗未能改善总生存期，且度伐利尤单抗加替西木单抗也并未为所有受试者提供总生存期益处[37]。

这些研究的详细结果将使临床医生能够全面评估在抗 PD-1/PD-L1 治疗中加入抗 CTLA-4 治疗的作用。

4.2　化疗与免疫治疗的联合或序贯治疗

KEYNOTE-040 试验、CHECKMATE-141 试验和 KEYNOTE-048 试验的结果皆显示：与标准治疗相比，抗 PD-1 治疗未能使无进展生存期（PFS）延长，但使总生存期（OS）更长。这一结果不能仅通过少部分患者因免疫治疗获得长期缓解来解释。另一个可能的因素是抗 PD-1 治疗可增强患者对化疗的敏感性。实际上，已有报道称免疫治疗后患者对化疗的反应增强。二线治疗的这种影响可以通过累积无进展生存期（PFS2）来评估，PFS2 定义为从随机分组到下一线治疗出现客观性肿瘤进展的时间或到因任何原因死亡的时间[38]。KEYNOTE-048 试验的事后分析研究了总人群、CPS ≥ 1 和 CPS ≥ 20 人群的 PFS2。结果显示：与 EXTREME 方案比较，在 CPS ≥ 1 和 CPS ≥ 20 人群中，接受帕博利珠单抗单药治疗的患者有更长的中位 PFS2；而接受帕博利珠单抗加化疗的患者，与 EXTREME 方案相比，在总人群、CPS ≥ 1 和 CPS ≥ 20 人群中也观察到更长的 PFS2[38]。这一结果表明，早期接受抗 PD-1 治疗可能通过改变肿瘤微环境，增强患者对后续治疗的敏感性。这些发现支持在一线治疗中优先使用抗 PD-1 药物。然而，仍需要通过前瞻性临床试验、转化性研究以及临床前研究进一步探索，以确定最有效的治疗方案和治疗顺序。

5　结论

PD-1 抑制剂已在复发/转移性头颈部鳞状细胞癌中显著改善了患者的总生存期，并且具有良好的耐受性。帕博利珠单抗获批作为一线治疗方案，可单药使用或与化疗联合使用，其选择基于联合阳性评分（CPS）评估的 PD-L1 表达水平。纳武利尤单抗被批准用于铂类治疗失败后的二线治疗。治疗方案的选择应以患者的个体情况为核心，进行全面评估和决策。相关的治疗推荐总结见图 2-2。铂类治疗失败患者：对于过去 6 个月内接受过铂类化疗的患者，可选择纳武利尤单抗或帕博利珠单抗。铂类敏感患者：治疗决策应以 CPS 水平为指导。如未进

第 2 章　头颈部肿瘤免疫治疗临床开发中的药物靶点与策略　47

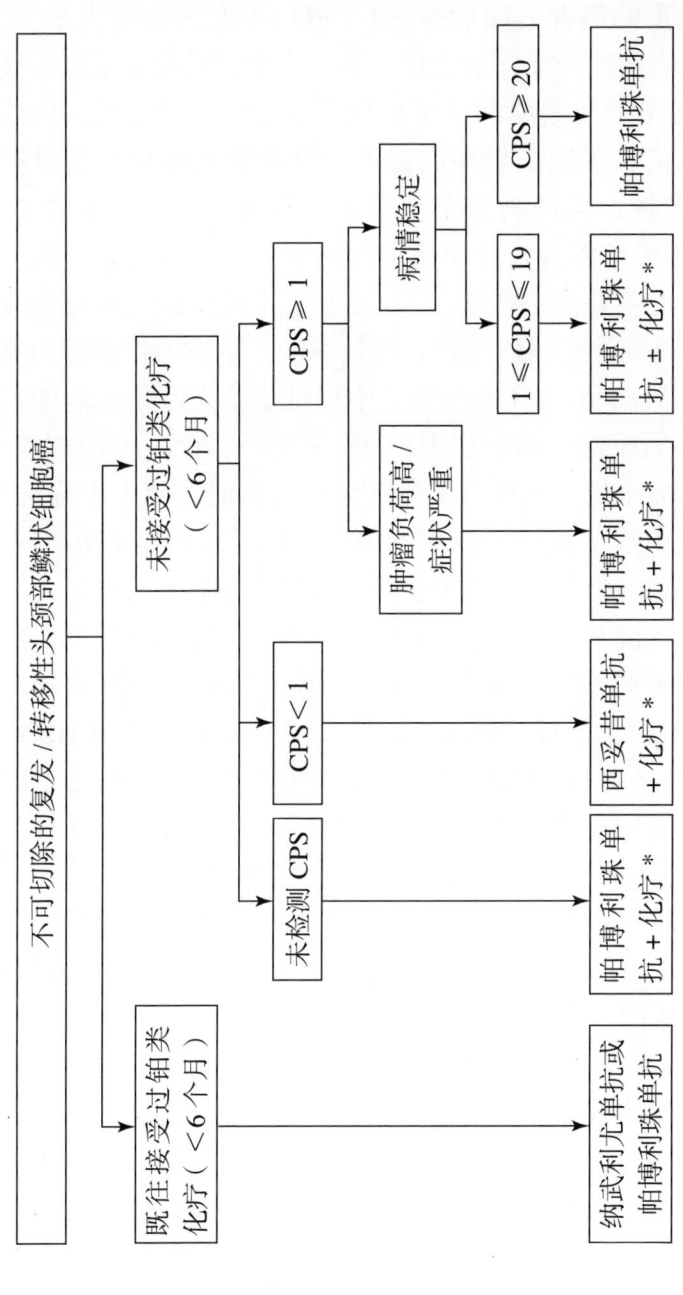

图 2-2　复发/转移性头颈部鳞状细胞癌的治疗选择。CPS：联合阳性评分

*铂类化疗

行 CPS 检测：推荐帕博利珠单抗联合化疗。如 CPS＜1（约占患者总数的 15%）：铂类化疗联合西妥昔单抗仍然是标准治疗选择，特别适用于肿瘤负荷较重的患者。如 CPS≥1（PD-L1 表达为阳性）：需根据患者肿瘤负荷和症状进一步评估治疗方案。当肿瘤负荷较重和（或）症状严重时，应优先考虑帕博利珠单抗联合化疗，以使肿瘤快速缩小。而对于无症状或症状稳定、轻微的患者，肿瘤快速缩小并非目标。对于 CPS≥20 的患者，帕博利珠单抗单药治疗是合理选择；而 CPS 为 1~19 的患者，则需要综合讨论单药治疗与联合化疗的利弊，因为这两种治疗的生存获益差异尚不明确[2,6]。并发症及禁忌证：需充分考虑患者是否存在自身免疫性疾病或化疗相关禁忌证，这在治疗选择中具有重要作用。尽管抗 PD-1 治疗在部分患者中展现了令人印象深刻的长期疗效，但总缓解率仍偏低，多数患者的缓解率低于 20%。未来需要进一步的转化研究和临床研究来提高治疗缓解率，同时优化患者筛选策略。目前，临床实践中唯一被广泛使用的预测生物标志物是 PD-L1 表达水平，包括肿瘤突变负荷等的其他生物标志物仍处于研究阶段。

为进一步提高抗 PD-1 治疗在 R/M HNSCC 中的疗效，正在探索多种免疫检查点抑制剂（ICI）的联合治疗策略。然而，目前的随机试验显示，抗 PD-1/PD-L1 与抗 CTLA-4 的联合治疗未能在 R/M HNSCC 中显著改善 OS。此外，抗 PD-1 治疗与化疗的联合方案虽然显示出生存情况和缓解率的有限提升，但与单纯化疗相比，其获益程度相当。因此，未来研究应关注于优化治疗顺序及治疗持续时间的新策略。

当疾病进展时，一些临床稳定的患者仍可能从继续使用同一 ICI 治疗中获益。对于少量局部进展（寡进展）的患者，立体定向放射治疗或其他局部治疗可能使更换系统性治疗方案的需求延缓，同时改善免疫治疗的效果。此外，一线使用抗 PD-1 治疗可能通过改变肿瘤微环境，提高肿瘤对后续化疗的敏感性。再挑战策略（在因疾病进展或不良反应停止治疗后重新使用相同或其他 ICI）值得进一步研究[39]。也有研究正在评估将 ICI 用于针对头颈部肿瘤早期阶段的治愈性策略中。在局部晚期疾病中，ICI 可作为针对高风险患者的治疗强化的手段，也可作为以减少化疗或放疗毒性为目标的治疗弱化的手段。这些新兴策略将为优化治疗提供新的可能性，其进展将在后续章节中详细讨论。

原文致谢　The authors wish to thank Aileen Eiszele for writing and editorial assistance.

原文符合伦理标准相关声明

Disclosure of Potential Conflicts of Interest　Athénaïs van der Elst: no disclosure.
Jean-Pascal Machiels: Advisory board member or speaker with honoraria (managed by my Institution): Pfizer, Roche, Astra/Zeneca, Bayer, Innate, Merck Serono, Boerhinger, BMS, Novartis, Janssen, Incyte, Cue Biopharma, ALX Oncology, iTEOS, eTheRNA, NEKTAR…
Travel expenses: Amgen, BMS, Pfizer, MSD.
Data safety monitoring board with honoraria: Psioxus.
Institutional conflict of interest (Funding to institution for research support): all companies.
Uncompensated advisory role: MSD.

Informed Consent　Not applicable.

参考文献

1. Bray F, Ferlay J, Soerjomataram I et al (2018) Global cancer statistics 2018: GLOBOCAN estimates of incidence and mortality worldwide for 36 cancers in 185 countries. CA Cancer J Clin 68:394-424. https://doi.org/10.3322/caac.21492
2. Machiels J-P, Leemans CR, Golusinski W et al (2020) Squamous cell carcinoma of the oral cavity, larynx, oropharynx and hypopharynx: EHNS-ESMO-ESTRO clinical practice guidelines for diagnosis, treatment and follow-up. Ann Oncol 31:1462-1475. https://doi.org/10.1016/j.annonc.2020.07.011
3. de Martel C, Georges D, Bray F et al (2020) Global burden of cancer attributable to infections in 2018: a worldwide incidence analysis. Lancet Glob Health 8:e180-e190. https://doi.org/10.1016/S2214-109X(19)30488-7
4. Chow LQM (2020) Head and neck cancer. N Engl J Med 382:60-72. https://doi.org/10.1056/NEJMra1715715
5. Vermorken JB, Mesia R, Rivera F et al (2008) Platinum-based chemotherapy plus cetuximab in head and neck cancer. N Engl J Med 359:1116-1127. https://doi.org/10.1056/NEJMoa0802656
6. Burtness B, Harrington KJ, Greil R et al (2019) Pembrolizumab alone or with chemotherapy versus cetuximab with chemotherapy for recurrent or metastatic squamous cell carcinoma of the head and neck (KEYNOTE-048): a randomised, open-label, phase 3 study. Lancet 394:1915-1928. https://doi.org/10.1016/S0140-6736(19)32591-7
7. Rotte A (2019) Combination of CTLA-4 and PD-1 blockers for treatment of cancer. J Exp Clin Cancer Res. https://doi.org/10.1186/s13046-019-1259-z
8. Mehra R, Seiwert TY, Gupta S et al (2018) Efficacy and safety of pembrolizumab in recurrent/metastatic head and neck squamous cell carcinoma: pooled analyses after long-term follow-up in KEYNOTE-012. Br J Cancer 119:153-159. https://doi.org/10.1038/s41416-018-0131-9
9. Bauml J, Seiwert TY, Pfister DG et al (2017) Pembrolizumab for platinum- and cetuximab-refractory head and neck cancer: results from a single-arm, phase II study. J Clin Oncol 35:1542-1549. https://doi.org/10.1200/JCO.2016.70.1524
10. Cohen EEW, Soulières D, Le Tourneau C et al (2019) Pembrolizumab versus methotrexate, docetaxel, or cetuximab for recurrent or metastatic head-and-neck squamous cell carcinoma

(KEYNOTE-040): a randomised, open-label, phase 3 study. Lancet 393:156-167. https://doi.org/10.1016/S0140-6736(18)31999-8
11. Ferris RL, Blumenschein G Jr, Fayette J et al (2016) Nivolumab for recurrent squamous-cell carcinoma of the head and neck. N Engl J Med 375(19):1856-1867. https://doi.org/10.1056/NEJMoa1602252
12. Ferris RL, Blumenschein G Jr, Fayette J et al (2018) Nivolumab vs investigator's choice in recurrent or metastatic squamous cell carcinoma of the head and neck: 2-year long-term survival update of CheckMate 141 with analyses by tumor PD-L1 expression. Oral Oncol 81:45-51. https://doi.org/10.1016/j.oraloncology.2018.04.008
13. Harrington KJ, Ferris RL, Blumenschein G Jr et al (2017) Nivolumab versus standard, single-agent therapy of investigator's choice in recurrent or metastatic squamous cell carcinoma of the head and neck (CheckMate 141): health-related quality-of-life results from a randomised, phase 3 trial. Lancet Oncol 18:1104-1115. https://doi.org/10.1016/S1470-2045(17)30421-7
14. Harrington KJ, Soulières D, Le Tourneau C et al (2021) Quality of life with pembrolizumab for recurrent and/or metastatic head and neck squamous cell carcinoma: KEYNOTE-040. J Natl Cancer Inst 113:171-181. https://doi.org/10.1093/jnci/djaa063
15. Guigay J, Fayette J, Mesia R et al (2019) TPExtreme randomized trial: TPEx versus Extreme regimen in 1st line recurrent/metastatic head and neck squamous cell carcinoma (R/M HNSCC). J Clin Oncol 37:6002-6002. https://doi.org/10.1200/JCO.2019.37.15_suppl.6002
16. Hecht M, Hahn D, Wolber P et al (2020) Treatment response lowers tumor symptom burden in recurrent and/or metastatic head and neck cancer. BMC Cancer. https://doi.org/10.1186/s12885-020-07440-w
17. Oliveira TB, Mesía R, Falco A et al (2021) Defining the needs of patients with recurrent and/or metastatic head and neck cancer: an expert opinion. Crit Rev Oncol Hematol. https://doi.org/10.1016/j.critrevonc.2020.103200
18. European Medicines Agency (2019) Public Assessment Report, Keytruda. https://www.ema.europa.eu/en/documents/variation-report/keytruda-h-c-3820-ii-0065-epar-assessment-report-variation_en.pdf. Accessed 10 June 2021
19. Sun C, Mezzadra R, Schumacher TN (2018) Regulation and function of the PD-L1 checkpoint. Immunity 48:434-452. https://doi.org/10.1016/j.immuni.2018.03.014
20. Haddad R, Concha-Benavente F, Blumenschein G et al (2019) Nivolumab treatment beyond RECIST-defined progression in recurrent or metastatic squamous cell carcinoma of the head and neck in CheckMate 141: A subgroup analysis of a randomized phase 3 clinical trial. Cancer 125:3208-3218. https://doi.org/10.1002/cncr.32190
21. Gameiro SF, Ghasemi F, Barrett JW et al (2018) Treatment-naïve HPV+ head and neck cancers display a T-cell-inflamed phenotype distinct from their HPV- counterparts that has implications for immunotherapy. Onco Targets Ther. https://doi.org/10.1080/2162402X.2018.1498439
22. Cohen EEW, Bell RB, Bifulco CB et al (2019) The Society for Immunotherapy of Cancer consensus statement on immunotherapy for the treatment of squamous cell carcinoma of the head and neck (HNSCC). J Immunother Cancer. https://doi.org/10.1186/s40425-019-0662-5
23. Saba NF, Blumenschein G Jr, Guigay J et al (2019) Nivolumab versus investigator's choice in patients with recurrent or metastatic squamous cell carcinoma of the head and neck: efficacy and safety in CheckMate 141 by age. Oral Oncol 96:7-14. https://doi.org/10.1016/j.oraloncology.2019.06.017

24. Johnson DB, Sullivan RJ, Menzies AM (2017) Immune checkpoint inhibitors in challenging populations. Cancer 123:1904-1911. https://doi.org/10.1002/cncr.30642
25. Saâda-Bouzid E, Defaucheux C, Karabajakian A et al (2017) Hyperprogression during anti-PD-1/PD-L1 therapy in patients with recurrent and/or metastatic head and neck squamous cell carcinoma. Ann Oncol 28:1605-1611. https://doi.org/10.1093/annonc/mdx178
26. Karabajakian A, Garrivier T, Crozes C et al (2020) Hyperprogression and impact of tumor growth kinetics after PD1/PDL1 inhibition in head and neck squamous cell carcinoma. Oncotarget 11:1618-1628. https://doi.org/10.18632/oncotarget.27563
27. Park JH, Chun SH, Lee Y-G et al (2020) Hyperprogressive disease and its clinical impact in patients with recurrent and/or metastatic head and neck squamous cell carcinoma treated with immune-checkpoint inhibitors: Korean cancer study group HN 18-12. J Cancer Res Clin Oncol 146:3359-3369. https://doi.org/10.1007/s00432-020-03316-5
28. Economopoulou P, Anastasiou M, Papaxoinis G et al (2021) Patterns of response to immune checkpoint inhibitors in association with genomic and clinical features in patients with head and neck squamous cell carcinoma (HNSCC). Cancers. https://doi.org/10.3390/cancers13020286
29. Borcoman E, Kanjanapan Y, Champiat S et al (2019) Novel patterns of response under immunotherapy. Ann Oncol 30:385-396. https://doi.org/10.1093/annonc/mdz003
30. Martins F, Sofiya L, Sykiotis GP et al (2019) Adverse effects of immune-checkpoint inhibitors: epidemiology, management and surveillance. Nat Rev Clin Oncol 16:563-580. https://doi.org/10.1038/s41571-019-0218-0
31. Zandberg DP, Algazi AP, Jimeno A et al (2019) Durvalumab for recurrent or metastatic head and neck squamous cell carcinoma: results from a single-arm, phase II study in patients with ≥ 25% tumour cell PD-L1 expression who have progressed on platinum-based chemotherapy. Eu J Cancer 107:142-152. https://doi.org/10.1016/j.ejca.2018.11.015
32. Siu LL, Even C, Mesía R et al (2019) Safety and efficacy of durvalumab with or without tremelimumab in patients with PD-L1-low/negative recurrent or metastatic HNSCC: the phase 2 CONDOR randomized clinical trial. JAMA Oncol 5:195-203. https://doi.org/10.1001/jamaoncol.2018.4628
33. Ferris RL, Haddad R, Even C et al (2020) Durvalumab with or without tremelimumab in patients with recurrent or metastatic head and neck squamous cell carcinoma: EAGLE, a randomized, open-label phase III study. Ann Oncol 31:942-950. https://doi.org/10.1016/j.annonc.2020.04.001 Drug Targets and Strategies in the Clinical Development of Immunotherapy for Head
34. Haddad R, Gillison M, Ferris RL et al (2016) Double-blind, two-arm, phase 2 study of nivolumab (nivo) in combination with ipilimumab (ipi) versus nivo and ipi-placebo (PBO) as first-line (1L) therapy in patients (pts) with recurrent or metastatic squamous cell carcinoma of the head and neck (R/M SCCHN)—CheckMate 714. Ann Oncol. https://doi.org/10.1093/annonc/mdw376.69
35. Bristol Myers Squibb (2019) Bristol-Myers Squibb reports first quarter financial results. https://news.bms.com/news/corporate-financial/2019/Bristol-Myers-Squibb-Reports-First-Quarter-Financial-Results/default.aspx. Accessed 4 Aug 2021
36. Argiris A, Harrington K, Tahara M et al (2021) LBA36 Nivolumab (N) + ipilimumab (I) vs EXTREME as first-line (1L) treatment (tx) for recurrent/metastatic squamous cell carcinoma of the head and neck (R/M SCCHN): Final results of CheckMate 651. Ann Oncol 32:S1310-S1311. https://doi.org/10.1016/j.annonc.2021.08.2113
37. AstraZeneca PLC (2021) Update on KESTREL Phase III trial of imfinzi with or without

tremelimumab in the 1st-line treatment of recurrent or metastatic head and neck cancer. https://www.astrazeneca.com/media-centre/press-releases/2021/update-on-kestrel-phase-iii-trial-for-imfinzi. html. Accessed 4 Aug 2021
38. Harrington KJ, Rischin D, Greil R et al (2020) KEYNOTE-048: progression after the next line of therapy following pembrolizumab (P) or P plus chemotherapy (P+C) vs EXTREME (E) as first-line (1L) therapy for recurrent/metastatic (R/M) head and neck squamous cell carcinoma (HNSCC). J Clin Oncol. https://doi.org/10.1200/JCO.2020.38.15_suppl.6505
39. Inno A, Roviello G, Ghidini A et al (2021) Rechallenge of immune checkpoint inhibitors: a systematic review and meta-analysis. Crit Rev Oncol Hematol. https://doi.org/10.1016/j.critrevonc.2021.103434

第3章　免疫治疗在局部晚期鼻咽癌中的应用

Immunotherapy in Locally Advanced Nasopharyngeal Carcinoma

（Jun Ma, Yu-Pei Chen　著）

（田素青，刘伟　译）

摘要

随着免疫检查点抑制剂（ICI）在多种肿瘤治疗中取得巨大成功，免疫治疗已成为抗肿瘤新疗法开发的研究热点。鼻咽癌（NPC）具有一些独特的特性，使其成为免疫治疗的潜在适应证。对于局部晚期鼻咽癌（locally advanced nasopharyngeal carcinoma，LA-NPC），免疫治疗不仅可能成为一种有前景的治疗策略，进一步改善患者的预后，还可能被用来开发降强度治疗（de-intensification therapy），以减少治疗相关毒性并提高患者的依从性。目前，ICI 治疗、肿瘤疫苗和过继性 T 细胞治疗在 LA-NPC 中的应用正在被广泛探索。本章对免疫治疗在 LA-NPC 中的应用进行了概述，首先介绍了常见的肿瘤免疫治疗策略，讨论了免疫治疗在鼻咽癌中的适应证，以及免疫治疗与化疗和放疗联合应用的机制及可行性，之后重点介绍 ICI 治疗以及其他形式的免疫治疗（如肿瘤疫苗

原作者信息

J. Ma · Y.-P. Chen (✉)
Department of Radiation Oncology, State Key Laboratory of Oncology in South China, Collaborative Innovation Center for Cancer Medicine, Guangdong Key Laboratory of Nasopharyngeal Carcinoma Diagnosis and Therapy, Sun Yat-sen University Cancer Center, Guangzhou, People's Republic of China
e-mail: majun@sysucc.org.cn; chenyup1@sysucc.org.cn

和过继性 T 细胞治疗）在 LA-NPC 中的应用，特别关注最具前景的 ICI 疗法。

> **关键词**
>
> 过继性 T 细胞治疗·肿瘤疫苗·降强度治疗·免疫检查点抑制剂·免疫治疗·局部晚期鼻咽癌·预后

1 引言

尽管放疗技术和联合化疗方案已取得显著进展，但 LA-NPC 的预后仍然有待进一步改善[1]。在接受吉西他滨联合顺铂诱导化疗后同步放化疗这一标准治疗方案的患者中，仍有 15% 的 LA-NPC 患者面临治疗失败[2]。通过调动免疫系统抗击肿瘤，免疫治疗为进一步改善 LA-NPC 患者的预后提供了新的可能性[1]。肿瘤免疫治疗主要包括免疫检查点抑制剂（ICI）疗法、肿瘤疫苗、过继性 T 细胞治疗、单克隆抗体和细胞因子治疗。在这些策略中，ICI 疗法已在多种恶性肿瘤中取得突破性进展[3-7]。因此，其在 LA-NPC 治疗中的潜在应用近年来受到广泛关注。本章综述了免疫治疗在 LA-NPC 中的应用，并特别聚焦于最具前景的 ICI 疗法。

鼻咽癌（NPC）具备多种独特的生物学特性，使其成为免疫治疗的理想适应证。首先，NPC 是一种与 EB 病毒（Epstein-Barr virus, EBV）密切相关的肿瘤，表达正常组织中不存在的病毒蛋白。这些病毒蛋白可作为潜在的肿瘤相关抗原（tumor-associated antigen, TAA），诱导抗肿瘤免疫反应。其次，NPC 是一种起源于鼻咽黏膜的淋巴上皮瘤，表现出显著的非恶性淋巴细胞浸润[8-9]。此外，NPC 肿瘤细胞中 PD-L1 的表达水平显著上调（可达 90%）[10]，并且 PD-L1 高表达与患者的不良预后密切相关[11-13]。同样，癌微环境中 CTLA-4 的过表达也被证明是 NPC 患者生存率降低的独立预测因子[14]。综上所述，这些特性表明免疫治疗是 NPC 的一种新型且极具前景的治疗选择。

2 局部晚期鼻咽癌中免疫检查点抑制剂疗法的现状

免疫检查点抑制剂（ICI）在鼻咽癌（NPC）中的治疗效果最初在复发或转移性疾病患者中得到验证。多项关键性单臂临床试验显示，抗PD-1单克隆抗体在复发或转移性NPC患者中具有显著的临床疗效[15-17]。KEYNOTE-028 Ib期研究招募了27例既往标准治疗失败的不可切除或转移性NPC患者，这些患者的肿瘤细胞或肿瘤浸润性淋巴细胞中PD-L1表达水平≥1%。研究结果显示，总缓解率（ORR）为26%，1年总生存率（OS）为63%，1年无进展生存率（PFS）为33%[16]。在另一项Ⅱ期试验中，纳入了44例既往治疗的复发或转移性NPC患者，纳武利尤单抗的治疗结果显示，ORR为20%，1年OS为59%，1年PFS为19%[17]。此外，另有两项Ⅰ期单臂临床试验表明，卡瑞利珠单抗联合化疗在复发或转移性NPC患者中可进一步提高疗效[15]。基于这些令人鼓舞的研究结果，美国国家综合癌症网络（National Comprehensive Cancer Network，NCCN）2020年第1版（v. 1.2020）指南推荐纳武利尤单抗作为既往接受过治疗的复发或转移性NPC患者的二线治疗方案，推荐帕博利珠单抗作为既往接受过治疗的PD-L1阳性的复发或转移性NPC患者的二线治疗方案。

上述试验中ICI在复发或转移性NPC患者中显示出的临床活性，激发了肿瘤学家探索其在局部晚期鼻咽癌（LA-NPC）患者中的应用。关于ICI疗法在LA-NPC中的应用，主要有三个关键问题需要解答。首先，哪些患者适合参与评估ICI疗法的临床试验。根据美国国家癌症研究所组织的临床试验规划会议达成的共识，Ⅲ～ⅣA期的NPC患者（不包括T3N0~N1疾病）被定义为高危LA-NPC患者，适合参与ICI疗法临床试验，因为这部分患者的5年PFS约为70%[18]。此外，血浆EBV DNA可作为选择参与此类临床试验患者的有效生物标志物。对于标准治疗后血浆EBV DNA仍可检测的患者，也应考虑纳入试验。

基于上述会议的共识，目前有多项随机对照试验正在评估ICI联合化疗和放疗在高危LA-NPC患者中的疗效（表3-1）。一项Ⅲ期临床试验招募了442名高危LA-NPC患者，这些患者在完成同步放化疗（可伴随或不伴随诱导化疗）后 4~6 周内被随机分组，以评估卡瑞利珠单抗作为辅助治疗的疗效。另外一项Ⅲ期临床试验也在研究信迪利单抗用于整个诱导化疗及同步治疗的疗效。这两项试验的主要终点为 3 年 PFS，次要终点包括 3 年 OS、3 年无远处转移生存率和 3 年局部区域无复发生存率。这些试验的结果备受期待，可能为将 ICI 疗法纳入 LA-NPC 的标准治疗提供重要依据，同时也可揭示 ICI 疗法引入综合放化疗方案的最佳时机及其最佳治疗周期。

除了进一步改善患者预后外，肿瘤学家还对开发降强度治疗表现出浓厚兴趣，即以 ICI 疗法替代以顺铂为基础的同步化疗，从而降低治疗相关毒性并提高患者依从性。目前至少有三项相关临床试验正在进行（表 3-1）。一项Ⅱ期试验（NCT03383094）正在包括 LA-NPC 在内的局部晚期头颈部鳞状细胞癌患者中比较帕博利珠单抗联合同步放疗与标准同步放化疗的安全性和疗效。另一项单臂多中心Ⅱ期试验（NCT03984357）正在评估在整个同步及辅助治疗阶段纳武利尤单抗联合放疗的效果。此外，一项Ⅲ期多中心试验（NCT04907370）正在研究是否可以通过诱导、同步及辅助阶段用特瑞普利单抗替代顺铂化疗而不影响治疗效果。这些研究的最终结果将揭示在采用 ICI 疗法的情况下是否可以安全省略同步化疗。

来自其他肿瘤研究的经验表明，仅部分患者可能从 ICI 疗法中获益。因此，LA-NPC 中 ICI 疗法的一大挑战是识别哪些患者可能无法从 ICI 疗法中受益，以尽量减少毒性和经济负担。虽然一些免疫相关指标（如肿瘤微环境中淋巴细胞浸润状态及反映免疫检查点表达的免疫特征）在 NPC 患者中的预后价值已有报道[8, 19-20]，但目前尚无强有力证据支持这些免疫相关生物标志物或其他临床预后因子（如治疗前和治疗后的 EBV DNA 水平及其清除率）与 ICI 疗法反应之间的关联。由于样本量限制，这些探索性生物标志物分析的统计效能可能不足。因此，未来需要更大规模的研究来识别和验证能够筛选 ICI 疗法潜在获益患者的有效生物标志物。

表 3-1 评估局部晚期鼻咽癌免疫检查点抑制剂治疗有效性的正在进行的临床试验

研究设计	样本量	多中心	人群	试验方案	控制方案	注册号
常规放化疗加入免疫检查点抑制剂的研究						
Ⅲ期双臂	442	是	Ⅲ~ⅣA期（不包括T3～T4N0和T3N1）；GP方案后4~6周，给予以顺铂为基础的放化疗	• 辅助治疗：卡瑞利珠单抗×12个周期	观察	NCT03427827
Ⅲ期双臂	417	是	Ⅲ~ⅣA期（不包括T3～T4N0和T3N1）	• 诱导期：GP+信迪利单抗×3个周期； • 同步治疗：顺铂+信迪利单抗×3个周期+IMRT：70 Gy，6~7周	• 诱导期：GP×3个周期； • 同步治疗：顺铂×3个周期+IMRT：70 Gy，6~7周	NCT03700476
Ⅱ期单臂	46	是	ⅣA期；WHO Ⅱ/Ⅲ型	• 诱导期：GP+帕博利珠单抗×2个周期； • 同步治疗：帕博利珠单抗+顺铂+IMRT； • 辅助治疗：帕博利珠单抗 200 mg×12个周期	不适用（NA）	NCT03734809

（续表）

研究设计	样本量	多中心	人群	试验方案	控制方案	注册号
降强度研究						
Ⅱ期双臂	114	是	Ⅲ～ⅣB期（T1～T2N2～N3M0或T3～T4N0～N3M0）	同步治疗：帕博利珠单抗200 mg + IMRT：70 Gy，33～35次，6.5周；辅助治疗：帕博利珠单抗×17个周期	同步治疗：顺铂×3个周期 + IMRT：70 Gy，33～35次，6.5周	NCT03383094
Ⅱ期单臂	146	是	Ⅲ～ⅣA期（不包括T3～4N0和T3N1）包括NPC的HNSCC	诱导期：GP+纳武利尤单抗×3个周期；同步治疗：纳武利尤单抗360 mg + IMRT：70 Gy，33次，5次/周，每天1次；辅助治疗：纳武利尤单抗×6个周期	不适用	NCT03984357
Ⅲ期双臂	494	是	局部晚期鼻咽癌（T4N1，T1～T4N2～N3）	诱导期：GP+特瑞普利单抗×3个周期；同步治疗：特瑞普利单抗 + IMRT：70 Gy，33次，5次/周，每天1次；辅助治疗：特瑞普利单抗×11个周期	诱导期：GP+特瑞普利单抗×3个周期；同步治疗：特瑞普利单抗+顺铂×3个周期 + IMRT：70 Gy，33次，5次/周，每天1次；辅助治疗：特瑞普利单抗×11个周期	NCT04907370

IMRT：调强放疗；GP：顺铂-吉西他滨方案

3　局部晚期鼻咽癌的其他免疫治疗

除了免疫检查点抑制剂治疗，其他形式的免疫治疗（如肿瘤疫苗和过继性 T 细胞治疗）也正在被探索用于治疗局部晚期鼻咽癌患者。由于地方性鼻咽癌是一种与 EB 病毒相关的肿瘤，研究者开发了以病毒蛋白作为肿瘤相关抗原（TAA）来启动或增强抗肿瘤免疫反应的肿瘤疫苗平台。在 NPC 的肿瘤疫苗中，最常使用的病毒蛋白是 EB 病毒核抗原（Epstein-Barr nuclear antigen，EBNA）和潜伏膜蛋白（latent membrane protein，LMP）[21]。由于 EBNA1 蛋白的 C 端富含 CD4 表位，而 LMP2 蛋白富含 CD8 表位，研究者设计了一种编码 EBNA1 C 端与 LMP2 融合蛋白的重组痘病毒肿瘤疫苗。这种疫苗在两项 I 期临床试验中针对接受一线治疗后处于 EBV 阳性的 NPC 患者进行了评估。结果显示，该疫苗能够剂量依赖性地扩增 LMP2 或 EBNA1 特异性 T 淋巴细胞，证明其具有较高的免疫原性[22-23]。目前，这种疫苗的疗效正在一项 II 期试验（NCT01094405）中进一步评估，研究对象为在接受常规治疗后仍可检测到血浆 EBV DNA 的 NPC 患者。此外，其他肿瘤疫苗（如腺病毒-ΔLMP1-LMP2 转导树突细胞疫苗和基于 LMP2 蛋白肽的疫苗）也正在开发，以应用于 NPC 患者[24]。

将针对 EBV 的细胞毒性 T 细胞（CTL）或肿瘤浸润性淋巴细胞（TIL）进行过继性转移是 EBV 阳性 NPC 患者除肿瘤疫苗外的另一种潜在免疫治疗策略。在多项临床试验中，尤其是针对转移性或复发性 NPC 患者的试验中，这种策略的临床疗效已得到证实[25-27]。目前，多个临床试验正在进行中，以进一步验证这种治疗策略的疗效（表 3-2）。如果这些策略的疗效能够得到确认，将为 LA-NPC 患者提供更多治疗选择。此外，ICI 疗法与肿瘤疫苗或过继性 T 细胞治疗的联合可能是一种理想且前景广阔的策略，可增强肿瘤疫苗诱导的抗肿瘤免疫反应或转移 T 细胞介导的免疫反应。

表 3-2 评估局部晚期或复发性鼻咽癌的过继性 T 细胞治疗的临床试验

研究设计	样本量	多中心	人群	试验方案/试验细胞	控制方案	注册号
正在进行中的临床试验						
II 期双臂	116	否	T3~T4N1~N3M0 或任意 T，N2~N3M0；血浆 EB 病毒 DNA ≥ 4000 拷贝/ml	• 同步治疗：顺铂 × 3 个周期 + 放疗； • 辅助治疗：肿瘤浸润性淋巴细胞输注	同步治疗：顺铂 × 3 个周期	NCT02421640
I/II 期单臂	20	否	EB 病毒阳性恶性肿瘤，包括鼻咽癌	PD-1 敲除的 CTL + 氟达拉滨 + 环磷酰胺 + IL-2	不适用	NCT03044743
I 期单臂	14	否	复发或难治鼻咽癌；EB 病毒阳性	TGF-β 耐受的 DNR 和鼻咽癌特异性 CTL + 环磷酰胺 + 氟达拉滨	不适用	NCT02065362
I 期单臂	27	否	EBER 阳性鼻咽癌；二线铂类化疗失败，或不可手术且无法放疗的复发/转移性疾病	LMP2 抗原特异性 CTL	不适用	NCT03925896
III 期双臂	330	是	转移性或复发性无根治性治疗选择	吉西他滨（1000 mg/m²）+ 卡铂（第 1 天，第 8 天，第 15 天，每 4 周 1 周期 × 4 周期）+ 自体 EB 病毒特异性细胞毒性 T 细胞；对照组：吉西他滨（1000 mg/m²）+ 卡铂（第 1 天，第 8 天，第 15 天，每 4 周 1 周期 × 6 周期）	吉西他滨 + 卡铂（标准方案）	NCT02578641
II 期单臂	20	否	EB 病毒阳性复发或转移鼻咽癌；一线和二线治疗失败	EB 病毒特异性 TCR T 细胞	不适用	NCT03648697

4　结论

免疫治疗可能成为改善 LA-NPC 患者预后的重要治疗策略。通过针对肿瘤免疫循环各步骤中的不同调节因子，已经开发了多种肿瘤免疫治疗方法。对于 LA-NPC 患者，目前正在深入探索 ICI 治疗、肿瘤疫苗以及过继性 T 细胞治疗的应用前景。其中，最具潜力的 ICI 疗法不仅能够进一步改善患者预后，还可能为开发减毒治疗提供可能，从而降低治疗相关毒性并提高患者的治疗依从性。

然而，有关 ICI 在 LA-NPC 患者中的应用仍存在许多未解答的问题，需要通过更多高质量的临床试验进一步研究。肿瘤疫苗和过继性 T 细胞治疗可能为 LA-NPC 患者提供额外的治疗选择。此外，将 ICI 疗法与肿瘤疫苗或过继性 T 细胞治疗相结合，有望成为增强这些治疗策略疗效的一种创新且有前景的方法。

原文符合伦理标准相关声明

Disclosure of Potential Conflicts of Interest　The author(s) declare that they have no competing interests.

Informed Consent　Not applicable.

参考文献

1. Chen YP, Chan ATC, Le QT et al (2019) Nasopharyngeal carcinoma. Lancet 394:64-80. https://doi.org/10.1016/s0140-6736(19)30956-0
2. Zhang Y, Chen L, Hu GQ et al (2019) Gemcitabine and cisplatin induction chemotherapy in nasopharyngeal carcinoma. N Engl J Med 381:1124-1135. https://doi.org/10.1056/NEJMoa1905287
3. Almquist DR, Ahn DH, Bekaii-Saab TS (2020) The role of immune checkpoint inhibitors in colorectal adenocarcinoma. BioDrugs 34:349-362. https://doi.org/10.1007/s40259-020-00420-3
4. Lavacchi D, Pellegrini E, Palmieri VE et al (2020) Immune checkpoint inhibitors in the treatment of renal cancer: current state and future perspective. Int J Mol Sci. https://doi.org/10.3390/ijms21134691
5. Akinleye A, Rasool Z (2019) Immune checkpoint inhibitors of PD-L1 as cancer therapeutics. J Hematol Oncol. https://doi.org/10.1186/s13045-019-0779-5
6. Doroshow DB, Sanmamed MF, Hastings K et al (2019) Immunotherapy in non-small cell lung cancer: facts and hopes. Clin Cancer Res 25:4592-4602. https://doi.org/10.1158/1078-0432.Ccr-18-1538

7. Queirolo P, Boutros A, Tanda E et al (2019) Immune-checkpoint inhibitors for the treatment of metastatic melanoma: a model of cancer immunotherapy. Semin Cancer Biol 59:290-297. https://doi.org/10.1016/j.semcancer.2019.08.001
8. Wang YQ, Chen YP, Zhang Y et al (2018) Prognostic significance of tumor-infiltrating lymphocytes in nondisseminated nasopharyngeal carcinoma: a large-scale cohort study. Int J Cancer 142:2558-2566. https://doi.org/10.1002/ijc.31279
9. Ono T, Azuma K, Kawahara A et al (2018) Prognostic stratification of patients with nasopharyngeal carcinoma based on tumor immune microenvironment. Head Neck 40:2007-2019. https://doi.org/10.1002/hed.25189
10. Fang W, Zhang J, Hong S et al (2014) EBV-driven LMP1 and IFN-γ up-regulate PD-L1 in nasopharyngeal carcinoma: implications for oncotargeted therapy. Oncotarget 5:12189-12202. https://doi.org/10.18632/oncotarget.2608
11. Lee VHF, Lo AWI, Leung CY et al (2016) Correlation of PD-L1 expression of tumor cells with survival outcomes after radical intensity-modulated radiation therapy for non-metastatic nasopharyngeal carcinoma. PLoS One. https://doi.org/10.1371/journal.pone.0157969
12. Zhu Q, Cai MY, Chen CL et al (2017) Tumor cells PD-L1 expression as a favorable prognosis factor in nasopharyngeal carcinoma patients with pre-existing intratumor-infiltrating lymphocytes. Onco Targets Ther. https://doi.org/10.1080/2162402x.2017.1312240
13. Larbcharoensub N, Mahaprom K, Jiarpinitnun C et al (2018) Characterization of PD-L1 and PD-1 expression and CD8+ tumor-infiltrating lymphocyte in Epstein-Barr virus-associated nasopharyngeal carcinoma. Am J Clin Oncol 41:1204-1210. https://doi.org/10.1097/coc.0000000000000449
14. Huang PY, Guo SS, Zhang Y et al (2016) Tumor CTLA-4 overexpression predicts poor survival in patients with nasopharyngeal carcinoma. Oncotarget 7:13060-13068. https://doi.org/10.18632/oncotarget.7421
15. Fang W, Yang Y, Ma Y et al (2018) Camrelizumab (SHR-1210) alone or in combination with gemcitabine plus cisplatin for nasopharyngeal carcinoma: results from two single-arm, phase 1 trials. Lancet Oncol 19:1338-1350. https://doi.org/10.1016/s1470-2045(18)30495-9
16. Hsu C, Lee SH, Ejadi S et al (2017) Safety and antitumor activity of pembrolizumab in patients with programmed death-ligand 1-positive nasopharyngeal carcinoma: results of the KEYNOTE-028 study. J Clin Oncol 35:4050-4056. https://doi.org/10.1200/jco.2017.73.3675
17. Ma BBY, Lim WT, Goh BC et al (2018) Antitumor activity of nivolumab in recurrent and metastatic nasopharyngeal carcinoma: an international, multicenter study of the Mayo Clinic Phase 2 Consortium (NCI-9742). J Clin Oncol 36:1412-1418. https://doi.org/10.1200/jco.2017.77.0388
18. Le QT, Colevas AD, O'Sullivan B et al (2019) Current treatment landscape of nasopharyngeal carcinoma and potential trials evaluating the value of immunotherapy. J Natl Cancer Inst 111:655-663. https://doi.org/10.1093/jnci/djz044
19. Wang YQ, Zhang Y, Jiang W et al (2019) Development and validation of an immune checkpoint-based signature to predict prognosis in nasopharyngeal carcinoma using computational pathology analysis. J Immunother Cancer. https://doi.org/10.1186/s40425-019-0752-4
20. Wang YQ, Chen L, Mao YP et al (2020) Prognostic value of immune score in nasopharyngeal carcinoma using digital pathology. J Immunother Cancer. https://doi.org/10.1136/jitc-2019-000334

21. Cao Y (2017) EBV based cancer prevention and therapy in nasopharyngeal carcinoma. NPJ Precis Oncol. https://doi.org/10.1038/s41698-017-0018-x
22. Taylor GS, Jia H, Harrington K et al (2014) A recombinant modified vaccinia ankara vaccine encoding Epstein-Barr Virus (EBV) target antigens: a phase I trial in UK patients with EBV-positive cancer. Clin Cancer Res 20:5009-5022. https://doi.org/10.1158/1078-0432.Ccr-14-1122-t
23. Hui EP, Taylor GS, Jia H et al (2013) Phase I trial of recombinant modified vaccinia ankara encoding Epstein-Barr viral tumor antigens in nasopharyngeal carcinoma patients. Cancer Res 73:1676-1688. https://doi.org/10.1158/0008-5472. Can-12-2448
24. Chia WK, Wang WW, Teo M et al (2012) A phase II study evaluating the safety and efficacy of an adenovirus-ΔLMP1-LMP2 transduced dendritic cell vaccine in patients with advanced metastatic nasopharyngeal carcinoma. Ann Oncol 23:997-1005. https://doi.org/10.1093/annonc/mdr341
25. Louis CU, Straathof K, Bollard CM et al (2010) Adoptive transfer of EBV-specific T cells results in sustained clinical responses in patients with locoregional nasopharyngeal carcinoma. J Immunother 33:983-990. https://doi.org/10.1097/CJI.0b013e3181f3cbf4
26. Chia WK, Teo M, Wang WW et al (2014) Adoptive T-cell transfer and chemotherapy in the first-line treatment of metastatic and/or locally recurrent nasopharyngeal carcinoma. Mol Ther 22:132-139. https://doi.org/10.1038/mt.2013.242
27. Li J, Chen QY, He J et al (2015) Phase I trial of adoptively transferred tumor-infiltrating lymphocyte immunotherapy following concurrent chemoradiotherapy in patients with locoregionally advanced nasopharyngeal carcinoma. Onco Targets Ther. https://doi.org/10.4161/23723556.2014.976507

第 4 章　免疫治疗在复发 / 转移性鼻咽癌中的应用

Immunotherapy in Recurrent and Metastatic Nasopharyngeal Carcinoma

（Brigette B. Y. Ma, Anthony T. C. Chan　著）

（李涛，雷润宏　译）

摘要

过去五年，鼻咽癌（nasopharyngeal carcinoma，NPC）免疫治疗领域迎来了重要的复兴，这主要得益于免疫检查点抑制剂在复发 / 转移性鼻咽癌（R/M NPC）治疗中的成功应用。在过去的二十年中，针对 EB 病毒和非针对 EB 病毒的免疫治疗策略已在早期临床试验中进行了评估。多项 II 期研究表明，在铂类耐药患者中，PD-1 抗体单药治疗具有显著的临床疗效。最近，三项双盲安慰剂对照的 III 期研究显示，在 R/M NPC 的一线治疗中，PD-1 抗体与铂类化疗联合使用能够显著改善治疗结局，使免疫治疗成为鼻咽癌的主流治疗选择之一。本章重点探讨 PD-1 抗体在鼻咽癌姑息治疗中的临床作用及意义。

关键词

吉西他滨 · 转移性 · 鼻咽癌 · 铂类药物 · PD-1 及 PD-1 抗体 · 复发

原作者信息

B. Y. Ma (✉) · A. T. C. Chan
State Key Laboratory of Translational Oncology, Department of Clinical Oncology, Sir YK Pao Centre for Cancer Hong Kong Cancer Institute, The Charlie Lee Precision Immunotherapy Program, The Chinese University of Hong Kong, Hong Kong SAR, China
e-mail: brigette@clo.cuhk.edu.hk

1　引言

非角化型鼻咽癌（nasopharyngeal carcinoma, NPC）是流行地区最常见的鼻咽癌亚型，与 EB 病毒（EBV）感染密切相关。在 AJCC 分期Ⅰ~Ⅱ期患者中，鼻咽癌主要采用单纯放疗（RT）；而对于Ⅲ~ⅣA 期以及某些高风险的Ⅱ期患者，则通常采用同步放化疗（concurrent chemoradiotherapy, CRT）[1]。尽管调强放疗（intensity-modulated RT, IMRT）等现代三维放射治疗技术显著提高了疗效，鼻咽癌患者的 5 年远处复发率仍 15%~30%[2]。局部区域复发相对少见，在接受 IMRT 治疗的非转移性Ⅲ~Ⅳ期患者中，5 年局部区域失败率为 9%~24%[3]。对于那些无法接受治愈性治疗的广泛转移性鼻咽癌或复发性疾病患者，化疗是主要的治疗选择[4]。以铂类为基础的多药联合化疗在复发或转移性鼻咽癌一线姑息治疗中的中位总生存期为 11~28 个月，而中位无进展生存期为 7~10 个月，这一数据源于Ⅱ期和Ⅲ期临床研究[1-2, 5]。对于铂类耐药患者，采用单药化疗（如吉西他滨或卡培他滨）的中位进展时间仅为 5~7.5 个月[2]。尽管偶尔有报道显示，极少数对化疗高度敏感的患者或仅有少量胸部转移灶的患者可实现超过 5 年的长期缓解[6]，但绝大多数患者的预后依然不佳，因此迫切需要开发更有效的全身治疗方案。

关于 EBV 相关鼻咽癌免疫治疗的研究已历经近二十年，但直到最近五年随着免疫检查点抑制剂的问世，免疫治疗才逐渐被纳入标准治疗范畴[1]。针对鼻咽癌的免疫治疗通常分为两大类：针对 EBV 的免疫治疗和非针对 EBV 的免疫治疗。早期的免疫治疗研究以探索为主，重点开发靶向 EBV 潜伏抗原 [如 EBNA1 和（或）LMP1/LMP2] 的治疗性 EBV 特异性疫苗，以及在治疗抵抗性鼻咽癌患者中采用自体细胞毒性 T 细胞（CTL）[1]。近年来的临床试验扩展到了更新的细胞治疗策略，例如选择性靶向 EBV 相关肿瘤抗原的异体 CTL（如 tabelecleucel），或 CD137L 激动剂诱导的自体树突细胞加载 EBV 肽的疫苗（CD137L: DC-EBV-VAX）[1]。然而，除正在进行的 VANCE 研究（NCT02578641）外，这些针对 EBV 的免疫治疗研究尚未进入Ⅲ期临床阶段。VANCE 研究旨在比较含铂-吉西他滨方案联合或不联合自体 EBV 特异性 CTL 作为 R/M NPC 一线治疗的疗效（NCT02578641）。

相比之下，非针对 EBV 的免疫治疗的临床开发更为成熟，如靶向表皮生长因子受体（EGFR）和免疫检查点蛋白的单克隆抗体。一些最近报道的Ⅲ期临床试验结果可能对 R/M NPC 的治疗策略产生深远影响。其他治疗策略目前仍处于早期开发阶段，如针对免疫检查点蛋白的双特异性抗体、抗体-药物偶联物，以及基因工程改造的细胞疗法如嵌合抗原受体 T 细胞治疗和其他免疫效应细胞疗法等[1]。

2 免疫检查点抑制剂的发展

2.1 难治性疾病的治疗

全外显子测序和单细胞测序研究增进了我们对鼻咽癌免疫环境的理解[1,7-8]。鼻咽癌是一种免疫"热"（免疫活跃）肿瘤，肿瘤微环境抑制性显著，伴有衰竭的 CD8+ T 细胞和效应性 T 细胞浸润，这些细胞高表达抑制性免疫检查点蛋白，如 PD-L1、LAG-3、GAL-9-TIM-3、TIGIT 和 CTLA4[1,8]。多种针对 PD-1 其配体（PD-L1）的单克隆抗体已在复发/转移性鼻咽癌的一线或后续治疗中通过Ⅰ/Ⅱ期和（或）Ⅲ期研究进行评估[1]。其中针对 PD-1 的单抗（PD1-Ab）包括帕博利珠单抗[9]、纳武利尤单抗[10]、卡瑞利珠单抗（camrelizumab）[11-12]、特瑞普利单抗（toripalimab）[13-14]、替雷利珠单抗（tislelizumab）[15]、斯巴达珠单抗（spartalizumab）[16] 和信迪利单抗（sintilimab）（NCT03700476）；针对 PD-L1 的单抗（PDL1-Ab）包括阿替利珠单抗（atezolizumab）和度伐利尤单抗（NCT04447612）[17]。对Ⅰ/Ⅱ期试验的 PD1-Ab 进行汇总分析显示，用于铂类难治性 R/M NPC 患者时 PD1-Ab 单药治疗的客观缓解率约为 27%，一年 PFS 为 25%，一年 OS 为 61%[18]。PDL1-Ab 的疗效尚未正式报道，关于阿替利珠单抗的一项Ⅰ/Ⅱ期篮式试验（basket trial）的早期报告显示，它在难治性 NPC 治疗中的活性有限[17]。

有两项随机试验在铂类耐药的 R/M NPC 患者中比较了 PD1-Ab 单药治疗与化疗（如卡培他滨、吉西他滨或紫杉类药物）的效果，其研究结果已完整报告[16]，也已作为会议摘要发表[19]。在一项随机Ⅱ期研究中，122例在一线铂类化疗后进展的患者以2∶1比例随机分组，接受斯巴达珠单抗治疗或化疗（单药或多药联合）。尽管该研究设计并非旨在检测生存差异，但趋势显示化疗组在中位无进展生存期（6.6个月对比1.9个月，$P=0.915$）和总缓解率（35%对比17.1%）方面优于免疫治疗组。然而，斯巴达珠单抗组在中位缓解持续时间（10.2个月对比5.7个月）和中位总生存期（25.2个月对比15.5个月）方面优于化疗组。KEYNOTE-122（NCT02611960）Ⅲ期试验是另一项随机研究，旨在检测总生存期差异。233例患者以1∶1比例随机分组，接受帕博利珠单抗治疗（200 mg每3周1次），或接受医生选择的单药化疗，直至疾病进展。结果显示该研究未达到总生存期的主要终点，帕博利珠单抗组和化疗组的中位总生存期分别为17.2个月和15.3个月（HR=0.90，95%CI：0.67~1.19，$P=0.22$）；中位无进展生存期分别为4.1个月和5.5个月（HR=1.28，95%CI：0.94~1.75）。两组在总缓解率（21.4%对比23.3%）、疾病控制率（50.4%对比63.8%）和缓解持续时间（12个月对比13.1个月）方面均无显著差异。亚组分析显示，不同年龄组和化疗方案之间的总生存期HR相似，但在地理分布上存在差异——在中国（包括香港和台湾）入组的患者中，帕博利珠单抗治疗组的总生存期有数值上的改善（$n=68$；HR=0.55；95%CI：0.31~0.96）。总体而言，斯巴达珠单抗研究和KEYNOTE-122研究均为阴性结果，因此化疗仍然是铂类耐药鼻咽癌患者的主要治疗选择。然而，这些研究表明，少数患者可能对PD1-Ab单药治疗产生持久反应，但目前尚无明确的预测生物标志物来识别这些患者。当前的研究重点是将PD1-Ab与化疗、靶向治疗或其他免疫检查点抑制剂联合使用，以进一步提高疗效[20]。

2.2 免疫检查点抑制剂的联合疗法

在R/M NPC的一线治疗中，基于铂类-吉西他滨的化疗方案被广泛使用。这一方案源于标志性的Ⅲ期GEM20110714研究，其结果显示该方案在缓解率和无进展生存期方面优于顺铂联合5-FU[5]。在一项Ⅰ/Ⅱ期卡瑞利珠单抗研究中，23例患者接受了卡瑞利珠单抗联合铂类-吉西他滨的治疗。结果显示，总缓解率为91%（95%CI：72%~97%），

1年PFS为61%。87%的患者出现了3级或更高级别的不良反应（主要为骨髓抑制和低钠血症），但未发生治疗相关的死亡事件[11]。基于这一结果，多个Ⅲ期研究比较了含或不含PD1-Ab的铂类-吉西他滨方案，相关结果将在下文讨论。

PD-1和CTLA-4的双重抑制作用已在一项Ⅱ期研究（NCT03097939）中进行评估，已报告初步结果。该研究纳入了在R/M NPC中经历过一线治疗失败的患者，评估了纳武利尤单抗联合伊匹木单抗的疗效。在40名接受治疗的患者中，总缓解率为30%，中位缓解持续时间为5.9个月。10%的患者报告了3~4级治疗相关的自身免疫反应或其他不良事件，包括低肾上腺功能症、肺炎和重症肌无力。

此外，以PD1-Ab为基础的联合免疫治疗正在进行多个早期阶段的临床试验，这些试验包括靶向其他免疫检查点蛋白的双特异性抗体、细胞毒性T细胞治疗、表观遗传调控剂（如组蛋白去乙酰化酶抑制剂）以及血管内皮生长因子受体酪氨酸激酶抑制剂。这些试验旨在探索新的联合治疗策略，以进一步提高疗效。

2.3 一线治疗中免疫检查点抑制剂的应用

由中国大陆制药公司赞助的三项Ⅲ期随机安慰剂对照试验的初步结果最近已被报道，研究均使用PD1-Ab，包括特瑞普利单抗、卡瑞利珠单抗和替雷利珠单抗（表4-1）[12,14,22]。这些研究针对的均是中国大陆和（或）东南亚地区的初治R/M NPC患者，研究设计、样本量及终点设置相似。患者按照1:1比例随机分组，接受约6个月的铂类-吉西他滨联合安慰剂或PD1-Ab治疗，随后在疾病进展前或最长2年的维持治疗阶段仅使用安慰剂或PD1-Ab。JUPITER-2试验和CAPTAIN-1st试验的早期分析结果显示，加入特瑞普利单抗或卡瑞利珠单抗的铂类-吉西他滨方案可使肿瘤进展或死亡风险几乎减半（JUPITER-2试验：HR=0.52，95%CI：0.36~0.74；CAPTAIN-1st 试验：HR=0.54，95%CI：0.39~0.76）[12,14]。其他终点（如总缓解率和缓解持续时间）也显示出类似的获益（见表4-1）。虽然JUPITER-2试验和CAPTAIN-1st试验的设计并未明确探讨总生存期（OS）差异，但在JUPITER-2试验中，免疫治疗联合化疗组显示出OS获益的趋势（HR=0.603，95%CI：

表 4-1　比较标准化疗与含抗 PD-1 抑制剂的试验方案在复发/转移性鼻咽癌一线治疗中效果的Ⅲ期临床试验

临床试验	JUPITER-2 [14]	CAPTAIN-1st [12]	RATIONALE 309 [22]
NCT 注册号	NCT03581786	NCT03707509	NCT03924986
地点	中国大陆，新加坡，中国台湾	中国大陆	中国大陆，中国台湾，泰国
样本量	289（HR = 0.67，双侧显著性水平 0.05，80% 统计功效）	263（HR = 0.63，单侧显著性水平 0.025，90% 统计功效）	263
主要终点	PFS	PFS	PFS
次要终点	ORR，DOR，DCR，OS，无进展生存率与总生存率，安全性	ORR，DCR，DOR，OS，安全性	ORR，PFS2，DOR
随访时间/月	17.4~17.9	15.6	15.5
PFS (IRC)	HR = 0.52，95%CI：0.36~0.74，P = 0.0003	HR = 0.54，95%CI：0.39~0.76，P = 0.0002	HR = 0.50，95%CI：0.37~0.68，9.6 个月对比 7.4 个月
OS	HR = 0.603，95%CI：0.364~0.997，P = 0.0462	HR = 0.67，95%CI：0.41~1.11	HR = 0.60，95%CI：0.35~1.01
ORR (IRC)			NA
• 试验组	77.4%	88.1%	
• 对照组	66.4%	80.6%	
中位缓解持续时间			NA
• 试验组	10.0 个月	9.9 个月	
• 对照组	5.7 个月	5.7 个月	
HR (95% CI)	HR = 0.50，95%CI：0.33~0.78	HR = 0.48，95%CI：0.34~0.68	

IRC：独立审查委员会；HR：风险比；PFS：无进展生存期；OS：总生存期；ORR：客观缓解率（objective response rate）；DOR：缓解持续时间；DCR：疾病控制率

0.364~0.9997，P=0.0462）。两组的 3~4 级治疗相关不良事件发生率相近。第三项研究是 RATIONALE-309 试验，使用替雷利珠单抗；研究赞助方的新闻稿中提到试验达到了 PFS 的主要终点，但具体数据尚未正式公布。在已报告的亚组分析中，JUPITER-2 试验显示，所有临床亚组（如年龄、体能状态、复发/转移性疾病状态、肝肺转移及入组前的同步放化疗）均观察到 PFS 获益 [12, 14]。在 CAPTAIN-1st 试验中，器官转移数量为单个和姑息化疗史 ≤ 4 线的患者，从免疫治疗联合化疗中获益的可能性较低 [12]。随着 OS 数据的进一步成熟，这些研究可能对 R/M NPC 一线治疗的临床实践产生深远影响。未来待解决的问题包括：确定在诱导期免疫治疗联合化疗后的进展治疗中最佳的维持策略，确定维持治疗的最佳持续时间，以及在后续治疗中再挑战 PD1-Ab。

2.4 针对表皮生长因子受体的单克隆抗体

嵌合型表皮生长因子受体抗体西妥昔单抗最初被用于联合卡铂治疗 12 个月内铂类化疗失败的 R/M NPC 患者 [23]。在接受治疗的 60 例患者中，总缓解率为 11.7%，中位进展时间仅为 2.7 个月。另一研究组评估了一种较为积极的多模式治疗方案，即在初治或复发的转移性 NPC 患者中，西妥昔单抗联合顺铂和多西他赛作为诱导治疗，随后对局部区域病灶进行同步化疗、西妥昔单抗和 IMRT 治疗，最后以口服卡培他滨维持治疗直至疾病进展 [24]。在诱导治疗期间，39.5% 的患者出现 3~4 级白细胞减少症，14% 出现发热性中性粒细胞减少症；在 IMRT 期间，23.5% 的患者发生 3~4 级皮炎。目前，该治疗策略的 Ⅲ 期验证试验正在进行（NCT02633176）。

3 PD1-Ab 的预测生物标志物

PD-L1 表达（以 CPS 评估）、治疗前后血浆 EBV DNA 水平、肿瘤突变负荷和基因特征（gene signature）等预测生物标志物已在接受 PD1-Ab 单药治疗或 PD1-Ab 联合化疗的 R/M NPC 患者中被评估。然而，这些标志物尚未准备好在日常实践中用于选择 PD1-Ab 治疗的患者。关于 PD-L1 表达与 PD1-Ab 疗效之间的关系，证据存在矛盾。在纳武利尤单抗和特瑞普利单抗的 Ⅱ 期单臂研究中，观察到一个无统计学显著性的趋势，即 PD-L1 表达水平与客观缓解率的增加相关 [10, 13]。然而，在 KEYNOTE-122 研究中，使用 CPS 评估 PD-L1 表达时，CPS＜10 或 ≥10 均未预测帕博利珠单抗对 OS 的获益。反而，CPS＜10 的患者从帕博利珠单抗治疗中获益较多（HR=0.58，95%CI：0.39~0.87）[19]。在Ⅲ期 JUPITER-2 研究的一线试验中，无论肿瘤细胞或免疫细胞的 PD-L1 表达如何，特瑞普利单抗联合化疗均显示 PFS 获益[14]。有趣的是，与 KEYNOTE-122 中的观察结果类似，JUPITER-2 研究也发现，在 PFS 方面，与 PD-L1 表达阳性（≥1%）的患者（HR=0.59，95%CI：0.388~0.893）相比，PD-L1 表达阴性的患者（HR=0.35，95%CI：0.153~0.808）似乎获得了更大的 PFS 增益，尽管在 JUPITER-2 研究中只有 15%（n=45）的患者 PD-L1 表达为阴性[14]。

血浆 EBV DNA 可通过定量 PCR 在超过 95% 的 R/M NPC 患者中检测到，是 NPC 的重要预后因素[1]。在 CAPTAIN-1st 研究中，初始诱导卡瑞利珠单抗联合化疗后血浆 EBV DNA 变为不可检测的患者，其 PFS 增益更大（HR=0.37，95%CI：0.22~0.63，P=0.0001）[12]。其他因素如肿瘤突变负荷和基因特征也被评估，但尚需在更大队列中验证[13]。

4　结论

R/M NPC 患者的预后正在改善，这得益于系统性治疗药物不断扩展，支持治疗措施改善，对少量转移灶患者应用局部消融治疗，以及近年来抗 PD-1 免疫治疗在一线姑息治疗中的发展。在Ⅲ期临床试验中，PD1-Ab 联合铂类-吉西他滨耐受性良好。化疗仍是铂类耐药患者后续治疗的主要选择，因为随机研究未能证明单用 PD1-Ab 优于化疗。尽管部分接受 PD1-Ab 单药治疗的患者可能会产生持久缓解，但目前尚无可靠的生物标志物来识别这些患者。因此，联合治疗方案可能会成为未来研究的重点。

原文致谢　This chapter is dedicated to the memory of the late Mr. M.C. Tsui, a keen marathon runner and was the first patient enrolled into the NCI-9742 study. We would like to acknowledge The Charlie Lee Charitable Foundation which has supported this work in part through the Precision Immunotherapy Program, The Chinese University of Hong Kong.

原文符合伦理标准相关声明

Disclosure of Potential Conflicts of Interests B.B.Y.M. is an advisory board member and receives speaker's honoraria from Bristol Myers Squibb, Merck Serono, MSD and Novartis and is a consultant for Y-Biologics and Viracta Therapeutics, Inc.

A.T.C.C. receives research funding from Merck Serono, MSD and Pfizer and is an advisory board member for MSD and Tessa Therapeutics.

Informed Consent NA.

参考文献

1. Wong KCW, Hui EP, Lo KW et al (2021) Nasopharyngeal carcinoma: an evolving paradigm. Nat Rev Clin Oncol 18(11):679-695. https://doi.org/10.1038/s41571-021-00524-x
2. Lee AWM, Ma BBY, Ng WT, Chan ATC (2015) Management of nasopharyngeal carcinoma: current practice and future perspective. J Clin Oncol 33(29):3356-3364. https://doi.org/10.1200/JCO.2015.60.9347
3. Au KH, Ngan RKC, Ng AWY et al (2018) Treatment outcomes of nasopharyngeal carcinoma in modern era after intensity modulated radiotherapy (IMRT) in Hong Kong: a report of 3328 patients (HKNPCSG 1301 study). Oral Oncol 77:16-21. https://doi.org/10.1016/j.oraloncology.2017.12.004
4. Bossi P, Chan AT, Licitra L et al (2021) Nasopharyngeal carcinoma: ESMO-EURACAN clinical practice guidelines for diagnosis, treatment and follow-up (dagger). Ann Oncol 32(4):452-465. https://doi.org/10.1016/j.annonc.2020.12.007
5. Zhang L, Huang Y, Hong S et al (2016) Gemcitabine plus cisplatin versus fluorouracil plus cisplatin in recurrent or metastatic nasopharyngeal carcinoma: a multicentre, randomised, open-label, phase 3 trial. Lancet 388(10054):1883-1892. https://doi.org/10.1016/S0140-6736(16)31388-5
6. Pan CC, Lu J, Yu JR et al (2012) Challenges in the modification of the M1 stage of the TNM staging system for nasopharyngeal carcinoma: a study of 1027 cases and review of the literature. Exp Ther Med 4(2):334-338. https://doi.org/10.3892/etm.2012.584
7. Li YY, Chung GT, Lui VW et al (2017) Exome and genome sequencing of nasopharynx cancer identifies NF-kappaB pathway activating mutations. Nat Commun 8:14121. https://doi.org/10.1038/ncomms14121
8. Chen YP, Yin JH, Li WF et al (2020) Single-cell transcriptomics reveals regulators underlying immune cell diversity and immune subtypes associated with prognosis in nasopharyngeal carcinoma. Cell Res 30(11):1024-1042. https://doi.org/10.1038/s41422-020-0374-x
9. Hsu C, Lee SH, Ejadi S et al (2017) Safety and antitumor activity of pembrolizumab in patients with programmed death-ligand 1-positive nasopharyngeal carcinoma: results of the KEYNOTE-028 study. J Clin Oncol 35(36):4050-4056. https://doi.org/10.1200/JCO.2017.73.3675
10. Ma BBY, Lim WT, Goh BC et al (2018) Antitumor activity of nivolumab in recurrent and metastatic nasopharyngeal carcinoma: an international, multicenter study of the Mayo Clinic Phase 2 Consortium (NCI-9742). J Clin Oncol 36(14):1412-1418. https://doi.org/10.1200/JCO.2017.77.0388
11. Fang W, Yang Y, Ma Y et al (2018) Camrelizumab (SHR-1210) alone or in combination with gemcitabine plus cisplatin for nasopharyngeal carcinoma: results from two single-arm, phase 1

trials. Lancet Oncol 19(10):1338-1350. https://doi.org/10.1016/S1470-2045(18)30495-9
12. Yang Y, Qu S, Li J et al (2021) Camrelizumab versus placebo in combination with gemcitabine and cisplatin as first-line treatment for recurrent or metastatic nasopharyngeal carcinoma (CAPTAIN-1st): a multicentre, randomised, double-blind, phase 3 trial. Lancet Oncol 22(8):1162-1174. https://doi.org/10.1016/S1470-2045(21)00302-8
13. Wang FH, Wei XL, Feng J et al (2012) Efficacy, safety, and correlative biomarkers of toripalimab in previously treated recurrent or metastatic nasopharyngeal carcinoma: a phase II clinical trial (POLARIS-02). J Clin Oncol 39(7):704-712. https://doi.org/10.1200/JCO.20.02712
14. Mai HQ, Chen QY, Chen D et al (2021) Toripalimab or placebo plus chemotherapy as first-line treatment in advanced nasopharyngeal carcinoma: a multicenter randomized phase 3 trial. Nat Med 27(9):1536-1543. https://doi.org/10.1038/s41591-021-01444-0
15. Shen L, Guo J, Zhang Q et al (2020) Tislelizumab in Chinese patients with advanced solid tumors: an open-label, non-comparative, phase 1/2 study. J Immunother Cancer 8(1):e000437. https://doi.org/10.1136/jitc-2019-000437
16. Even C, Wang HM, Li SH et al (2021) Phase II, randomized study of spartalizumab (PDR001), an anti-PD-1 antibody, versus chemotherapy in patients with recurrent/metastatic nasopharyngeal cancer. Clin Cancer Res 27(23):6413-6423. https://doi.org/10.1158/1078-0432.CCR-21-0822
17. Shen L, Zhang L, Hu X et al (2018) Atezolizumab monotherapy in Chinese patients with locally advanced or metastatic solid tumors. Ann Oncol 29(Suppl_9):ix46. https://doi.org/10.1093/annonc/mdy432.006
18. Wang BC, Cao RB, Fu C et al (2020) The efficacy and safety of PD-1/PD-L1 inhibitors in patients with recurrent or metastatic nasopharyngeal carcinoma: a systematic review and meta-analysis. Oral Oncol 104:104640. https://doi.org/10.1016/j.oraloncology.2020.104640
19. Chan ATC, Lee VHF, Hong RL et al (2021) A phase III study of pembrolizumab (pembro) monotherapy vs chemotherapy (chemo) for platinum-pretreated, recurrent or metastatic (R/M) nasopharyngeal carcinoma (NPC). Ann Oncol 32:S786. https://doi.org/10.1016/j.annonc.2021.08.1268
20. Le QT, Colevas AD, O'Sullivan B et al (2019) Current treatment landscape of nasopharyngeal carcinoma and potential trials evaluating the value of immunotherapy. J Natl Cancer Inst 111(7):655-663. https://doi.org/10.1093/jnci/djz044
21. Kao H, Ang M, Ng QS et al (2020) Combination ipilimumab and nivolumab in recurrent/metastatic nasopharyngeal carcinoma (R/M NPC)—updated efficacy and safety analysis of NCT03097939. Ann Oncol 31(Suppl_6):S1347. https://doi.org/10.1016/j.annonc.2020.10.260
22. Z Li, Yang Y, Pan J.-j et al. (2022) RATIONALE-309: updated progression-free survival (PFS), PFS after next line of treatment, and overall survival from a phase 3 double-blind trial of tislelizumab versus placebo, plus chemotherapy, as first-line treatment for recurrent/metastatic nasopharyngeal cancer. J Clin Oncol 40(36_suppl):384950-384950
23. Chan ATC, Hsu MM, Goh BC et al (2005) Multicenter, phase II study of cetuximab in combination with carboplatin in patients with recurrent or metastatic nasopharyngeal carcinoma. J Clin Oncol 23(15):3568-3576. https://doi.org/10.1200/JCO.2005.02.147
24. Zhang M, Huang H, Li X et al (2020) Long-term survival of patients with chemotherapy-naive metastatic nasopharyngeal carcinoma receiving cetuximab plus docetaxel and cisplatin regimen. Front Oncol 10:1011. https://doi.org/10.3389/fonc.2020.01011

第5章 超越 PD-1/PD-L1 免疫检查点抑制剂：头颈部肿瘤的其他靶点与治疗方法

Beyond PD-1/PD-L1 Immune Checkpoint Inhibitors: Other Targets and Approaches for Head and Neck Cancer

（Niki Gavrielatou, Panagiota Economopoulou, Amanda Psyrri 著）
（茅芯慧，肖宇 译）

摘要

近年来，免疫治疗显著改变了头颈部肿瘤的治疗模式，已成为晚期疾病的标准治疗方案。然而，尽管最初大家充满热情，目前获批的针对程序性死亡受体1（PD-1）和程序性死亡受体配体1（PD-L1）免疫抑制通路的药物仅在少部分患者中显示了临床获益，复发患者的预后极差。在此背景下，研究者将重点转向其他免疫检查点分子，希望通过克服耐药性进一步优化免疫治疗的效果。日益增多的临床前证据表明，头颈部肿瘤微环境中存在多种免疫检查点的协同作用，这为临床研究联合抑制策略的疗效铺平了道路，目标是最大限度地增强宿主的抗肿瘤免疫反应。

原作者信息

N. Gavrielatou
Department of Pathology, Yale University School of Medicine, New Haven, CT, USA

P. Economopoulou · A. Psyrri (✉)
Department of Medicine, School of Medicine, National and Kapodistrian University of Athens, Athens, Greece
e-mail: psyrri237@yahoo.com

关键词

CTLA-4 · 头颈部肿瘤 · 免疫检查点 · 免疫治疗 · LAG-3 · PD-1 · PD-L1 · TIGIT

1　引言

头颈部肿瘤（HNC）是一类在病因学、组织学和预后方面具有异质性的肿瘤。鳞状分化是 HNC 最常见的组织学亚型，来源于口腔、喉、口咽、下咽及鼻旁窦黏膜的恶性肿瘤都被归类于 HNC 中。当前，HNC 是全球第八大常见肿瘤，发病率呈上升趋势，每年约新增 80 万例病例，死亡 40 万例[1-2]。吸烟、饮酒以及人乳头瘤病毒（HPV）感染是 HNC 发生的主要病因，其中，HPV 感染是发达国家新增口咽癌（OPC）的主要致病因素[3]。HPV 相关的肿瘤发生机制是通过 E6 和 E7 致癌蛋白分别使抑癌蛋白 p53 和 Rb 失活。HPV 阳性肿瘤具有独特的基因组特征，包括癌基因改变更频繁及 PIK3CA、PTEN、AKT1、RICTOR、mTOR、AKT2 和 PIK3R1 基因突变增加，而 TP53 突变则在 HPV 阴性肿瘤中更常见[4-5]。相比之下，烟草致癌主要通过形成 DNA 加合物导致复制缺陷及持续基因改变。与烟草相关的突变已在《癌症体细胞突变目录》（Catalogue for Somatic Mutations in Cancer, COSMIC）的突变特征 4（Mutational signature 4）中详细描述，这些突变表现为较高的肿瘤突变负荷，尤其在喉癌中更为明显[6]。

对于早期诊断的 HNC 患者，治愈率较高，5 年总生存率可达 90%。然而，大多数患者确诊时已是局部晚期，即使接受标准治疗，吸烟相关的 HNC 患者的 5 年生存率仅约 50%[7]；而对于 HPV 相关的 OPC，3 年总生存率可高达 82.4%（95%CI：77.2%~87.6%）[8]。对于晚期疾病，治疗通常需要由多学科团队制定多模式策略，包括手术、放疗、化疗和（或）免疫治疗，根据具体病例特点按照现行指南灵活组合[9]。近年来，复发或转移性头颈部肿瘤（R/M HNC）的治疗格局因免疫治疗的引入而发生了重大改变，这些治疗靶向 PD-1/PD-L1 免疫抑制通路，是对传统治疗手段的补充。如前面章节所述，目前两种靶向 PD-1 的单克隆抗体——纳武利尤单抗和帕博利珠单抗，已获得美国食品药品监督管理局（FDA）和欧洲药品管理局（EMA）的批准，用于 R/M HNC 的一线治疗及后线治疗。然而，尽管免疫治疗在这种侵袭性肿瘤的治疗中具有重要地位，R/M HNSCC 患者的总缓解率仍然较低，仅为 13.3%~18%，这一现状标明迫切需要开发可靠的预测生物标志物[10]。

抑制 PD-1/PD-L1 通路为目前 HNC 免疫检查点抑制药物的开发奠定了基础。然而，这些药物的疗效有限，说明迫切需要探索新的免疫调节靶点。本章节旨在全面梳理 HNC 中除 PD-1/PD-L1 通路以外的其他免疫检查点通路，这些通路作为新型抗肿瘤治疗策略的开发方向正在被研究。图 5-1 总结了目前在 HNC 领域具有临床研究意义的免疫治疗策略。

2 细胞毒性 T 淋巴细胞相关抗原 4（CTLA-4, CD152）

James Allison 发现 CTLA-4 是肿瘤免疫治疗领域的突破性进展，开启了肿瘤治疗的免疫学时代。CTLA-4 是一种免疫调节受体，与 PD-1 同属于免疫球蛋白超家族，主要在 CD4+、CD8+ T 细胞以及调节性 T 细胞（Treg）的细胞质内存在，通过内吞作用从细胞膜转移至细胞内囊泡[11]。CTLA-4 通过与抗原呈递细胞（APC）表面的配体 CD80（B7-1）和 CD86（B7-2）结合参与免疫抑制作用。与 CD28 相比，CTLA-4 与 CD80/CD86 的结合具有更高的亲和力和结合能力，表明 CTLA-4 对 CD28 共刺激通路起拮抗作用。在生理条件下，Treg 表达的 CTLA-4 通过竞争性抑制 CD28/B7 的相互作用，限制 APC 和 T 细胞的活性，从而维持免疫平衡。当炎症刺激 CD80/CD86 的表达增加时，这种抑制作用可能被克服。然而，在肿瘤微环境（tumor microenvironment, TME）中，Treg 异常浸润以及由肿瘤细胞分泌的转化生长因子 -β（TGF-β）诱导的 CTLA-4 过表达，导致持续的免疫抑制状态，从而帮助肿瘤细胞逃避宿主的抗肿瘤免疫反应[12]。

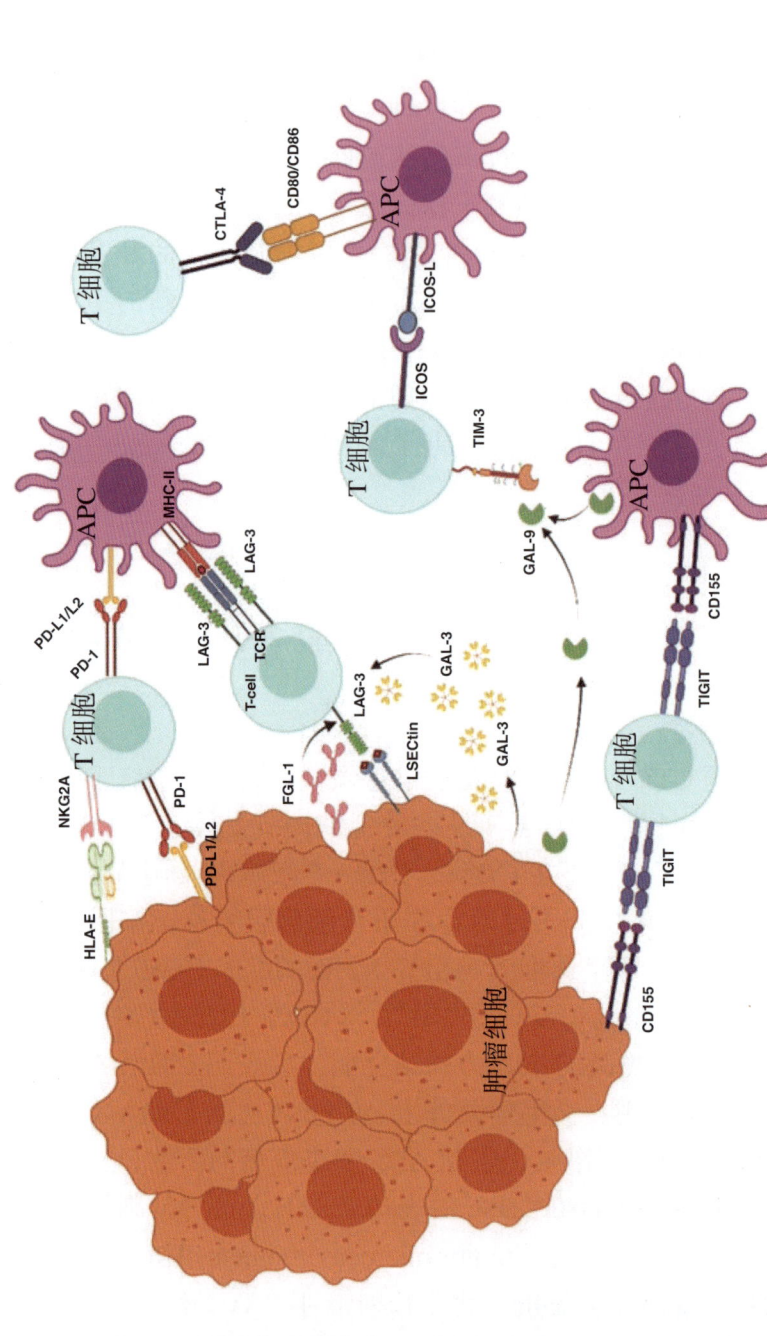

图 5-1 免疫检查点在头颈部肿瘤中的作用。HNC：头颈部肿瘤；PD-1：程序性死亡受体 1；PD-L1：程序性死亡受体配体 1；PD-L2：程序性死亡受体配体 2；APC：抗原呈递细胞；CTLA-4：细胞毒性 T 淋巴细胞相关抗原 4；LAG-3：淋巴细胞活化基因 3；FGL-1：纤维蛋白原样蛋白 1；GAL-3：半乳凝素 3；GAL-9：半乳凝素 9；LSECtin：肝和淋巴结窦状内皮细胞 C 型凝集素；ICOS：诱导性共刺激分子；ICOS-L：诱导性共刺激分子配体；TIM-3：T 细胞免疫球蛋白黏蛋白 3；TIGIT：T 细胞免疫球蛋白及免疫受体酪氨酸基抑制基序；TCR：T 细胞受体；HLA-E：人类白细胞抗原 E；NKG2A：NK 组 2 成员 A；MHC Ⅱ：主要组织相容性复合体 Ⅱ。本图通过 Biorender.com 绘制。

几项临床前研究揭示了 CTLA-4 在 HNC 中的重要生物学作用。Yu 等研究显示，与正常口腔黏膜相比，HNC 中 CTLA-4 的表达显著升高。研究还表明，CD8+/CTLA-4 比值高与较好的预后相关，而单独的 CD8+ 或 CTLA-4 表达未显示类似的独立预后价值。此外，CD8+/CTLA-4 比值与肿瘤微环境中免疫抑制型髓源性抑制细胞（MDSC）和 M2 型巨噬细胞的存在密切相关[13]。在免疫功能完整的 HNC 小鼠模型中，Pten/Tgfbr1 敲除小鼠 MDSC 和 M2 型巨噬细胞的水平显著升高，而 CTLA-4 抑制剂能够逆转这种现象，从而导致肿瘤缩小[13]。另一项研究中，在与烟草相关的 HNC 人类小鼠模型中 CTLA-4 抑制剂也引起了肿瘤退缩[14]。总体而言，这些研究表明 CTLA-4 在 HNC 的免疫抑制微环境中发挥关键作用，为通过抗 CTLA-4 治疗 HNC 提供了合理的理论支持。

CTLA-4 抑制剂已在多种恶性肿瘤中被评估，包括单药治疗和联合治疗。试验评估了两种完全人源化的抗 CTLA-4 单克隆抗体，即伊匹木单抗和替西木单抗，各研究结果并不相同，疗效在很大程度上取决于肿瘤类型的免疫原性。2011 年，伊匹木单抗成为首个被批准用于临床的免疫检查点抑制剂，最初用于治疗不可切除的Ⅲ期或Ⅳ期转移性黑色素瘤[15]。在头颈部肿瘤中，伊匹木单抗和替西木单抗也已被评估，但无论是单药治疗还是联合治疗，到目前为止的研究结果都不令人满意。CONDOR 研究是一项Ⅱ期临床试验，评估度伐利尤单抗单药、替西木单抗单药及两者联合作为 PD-L1 阴性（按 Ventana SP263 试验定义）的 R/M HNC 患者二线治疗的疗效，结果显示 ORR 在单药治疗组和联合治疗组皆未改善（度伐利尤单抗单药：9.2%，替西木单抗单药：1.6%，度伐利尤单抗与替西木单抗联合：7.8%）[16]。在Ⅲ期 EAGLE 试验中，736 例一线治疗失败的 R/M HNC 患者被随机分配接受以下三个治疗方案之一：度伐利尤单抗单药治疗，度伐利尤单抗与替西木单抗联合治疗，标准治疗（SoC），生存期分析显示，与标准治疗相比，无论是 PD-L1 抑制剂单药治疗（HR=0.88，95%CI：0.72~1.08，P=0.20）还是 PD-L1 抑制剂与 CTLA-4 抑制剂联合治疗（HR=1.04，95%CI：0.85~1.26，P=0.76），均未显著延长 OS[17]。Ⅲ期 KESTREL（NCT02551159）试验评估一线治疗的疗效，初治 R/M HNC 患者被随机分配接受以下三个治疗方案之一：度伐利尤单抗单药治疗，度伐利尤单抗与替西木单抗联合治疗，EXTREME 方案（西妥昔单抗方案 + 顺铂或卡铂 +5-FU）。尽管该研究的数据尚未正式发布，但最近该研究的赞助公司（AstraZeneca）宣布该研究未达到其主要终点，在度伐利尤单抗组 PD-L1 高表达患者中未观察到 OS 获益，在度伐利尤单抗联合替西木单抗组的总人群中也未观察到 OS 益处（次要终点）[18]。也有 II 期临床试验（NCT03693612）正在 PD-1/PD-L1 治疗失败的 HNC 患者中评估替西木单抗与 fladilimab（一种作为 ICOS 激动剂的人源化单抗）联合治疗的疗效。

另外两项在 R/M HNC 患者中评估伊匹木单抗与纳武利尤单抗联合治疗的试验结果同样令人失望。在 II 期 CHECKMATE-714 试验中，既往未接受治疗的患者和铂类耐药患者被随机分配接受纳武利尤单抗联合伊匹木单抗或纳武利尤单抗加安慰剂，初步公布的研究结果表明主要终点未达到。III 期 CHECKMATE-651 试验比较了纳武利尤单抗联合伊匹木单抗与 EXTREME 方案在一线治疗中的疗效[18]，关于该试验 Bristol Myers Squibb 在最近一份新闻稿中宣布，尽管纳武利尤单抗联合伊匹木单抗在 CPS ≥ 20 的患者中显示出清晰的 OS 正向趋势，但该研究未达到其主要终点。表 5-1 总结了关于 PD-1/PD-L1 通路之外其他免疫检查点抑制的临床试验，这些试验有些已经完成，有些正在进行。

译者注：尽管 CTLA-4 抑制剂在其他肿瘤中的研究显示出一定疗效，但在头颈部肿瘤中的临床试验结果并不理想。这可能与头颈部肿瘤特有的肿瘤微环境和较低的免疫原性有关。期待未来的研究集中于优化剂量、降低毒性、开发新的联合治疗策略，进一步探讨 CTLA-4 在头颈部肿瘤中的作用机制，以更好地利用其治疗潜力。

3 诱导性共刺激分子（ICOS, CD278）

诱导性共刺激分子（inducible T cell co-stimulator, ICOS）是 CD28/CTLA-4/B7 免疫球蛋白超家族的成员，其与 CTLA-4 和 CD28 在结构上相关，但表达模式和功能存在显著差异。除了调节 T 细胞的表达和功能外，ICOS 还在胸腺依赖性抗体生成和生发中心（germinal center, GC）反应中通过与其配体 ICOSL 的相互作用发挥关键作用。临床前研究表明，ICOS 能够独立于 CD28 信号促进 T 细胞增殖，并在调节 Th1/

表 5-1 头颈部肿瘤中关于除 PD-1/PD-L1 之外的免疫检查点抑制剂的临床试验

免疫检查点或其他	试验名称	NCT 注册号	临床分期	干预措施/组别	治疗方案	试验状态	结果
CTLA-4	CONDOR	NCT02319044	II	度伐利尤单抗/替西木单抗/度伐利尤单抗,替西木单抗	二线	已完成	ORR: 9.2%/1.6%/7.8%
	EAGLE	NCT02369874	III	度伐利尤单抗/度伐利尤单抗,替西木单抗/SoC	二线	已完成	ORR: 17.9%/18.2%/17.3%
	KESTREL	NCT02551159	III	度伐利尤单抗/度伐利尤单抗,替西木单抗/SoC	一线	已完成	结果待定
	N/A	NCT03693612	II	替西木单抗, feladilimab/SoC	二线	活跃,未招募	结果待定
	CheckMate 714	NCT02823574	II	纳武利尤单抗,伊匹木单抗/纳武利尤单抗,安慰剂	一线,二线	活跃,未招募	结果待定
	CheckMate 651	NCT02741570	III	纳武利尤单抗,伊匹木单抗/SoC	一线	活跃,未招募	结果待定
ICOS	INDUCE-3	NCT04128696	II/III	帕博利珠单抗, feladilimab/帕博利珠单抗,安慰剂	一线	活跃,未招募	结果待定
	INDUCE-4	NCT04428333	II/III	帕博利珠单抗, 5-FU-铂类化疗, feladilimab/帕博利珠单抗, 5-FU-铂类化疗,安慰剂	一线	活跃,未招募	结果待定
	N/A	NCT03251924	I/II	BMS-986226/BMS-986226, 纳武利尤单抗/BMS-986226, 伊匹木单抗	二线	活跃,未招募	结果待定
LAG-3	TACTI-002	NCT03625323	II	帕博利珠单抗, eftilagimod alpha	二线	招募中	ORR: 39% (DCR: 50%)

（续表）

免疫检查点或其他	试验名称	NCT注册号	临床分期	干预措施/组别	治疗方案	试验状态	结果
LAG-3	N/A	NCT04080804	Ⅱ	纳武利尤单抗，relatlimab/纳武利尤单抗，伊匹木单抗	新辅助治疗	招募中	结果待定
	N/A	NCT04326257	Ⅱ	纳武利尤单抗，relatlimab；纳武利尤单抗，伊匹木单抗	二线	招募中	结果待定
TIGIT	SKYSCRAPER-09	NCT04665843	Ⅱ	阿替利珠单抗，tiragolumab/阿替利珠单抗，安慰剂	一线	招募中	结果待定
IDO1	ECHO-202/KEYNOTE-037	NCT02178722	Ⅰ/Ⅱ	帕博利珠单抗，epacadostat	二线	已完成	ORR: 34% (DCR: 62%)
	ECHO-304/KEYNOTE-669	NCT03358472	Ⅲ	帕博利珠单抗，epacadostat/帕博利珠单抗/EXTREME	一线	活跃，未招募	结果待定
	ECHO-204	NCT02327078	Ⅰ/Ⅱ	纳武利尤单抗/epacadostat	二线	已完成	DCR: 70%
	ECHO-203	NCT02318277	Ⅰ/Ⅱ	度伐利尤单抗/epacadostat	二线	已完成	结果待定
	N/A	NCT03208959	Ⅰ	HTI-1090	二线	已完成	结果待定
	N/A	NCT03343613	Ⅰa/Ⅰb	LY3381916，LY3300054	二线	已终止	N/A
	N/A	NCT03854032	Ⅱ	linrodostat，纳武利尤单抗/纳武利尤单抗	新辅助治疗	招募中	结果待定

（续表）

免疫检查点或其他	试验名称	NCT注册号	临床分期	干预措施/组别	治疗方案	试验状态	结果
NKG2A	INTERLINK-1	NCT04590963	III	monalizumab，西妥昔单抗/西妥昔单抗，安慰剂	二线	招募中	结果待定
	N/A	NCT02643550	Ib/II	monalizumab，西妥昔单抗/monalizumab，西妥昔单抗，抗PD-1/PD-L1	二线	活跃，未招募	ORR: 27.5% (DCR: 37%)
	UPSTREAM	NCT03088059	II（基于生物标志物）	monalizumab/monalizumab，度伐利尤单抗/SoC	二线	招募中	结果待定
	N/A	NCT02331875	Ib/II	monalizumab	新辅助治疗	已终止	N/A
OX40	N/A	NCT02274155	I	MEDI6469	新辅助治疗	活跃，未招募	耐受性良好/↑免疫原性
	N/A	NCT03336606	I	MEDI0562	新辅助治疗	活跃，未招募	结果待定
	JAVELIN Medley	NCT02554812	Ib/II	阿维鲁单抗，PF-04518600/阿维鲁单抗，utomilumab, PF-04518600, CMP-001	多线	活跃，未招募	结果待定
VISTA	N/A	NCT02671955	I	onvatilimab	多线	已终止	N/A
	N/A	NCT02812875	I	CA-170	三线	已完成	结果待定
	N/A	NCT04475523	I	CI-8993	二线	招募中	结果待定

（续表）

免疫检查点或其他	试验名称	NCT注册号	临床分期	干预措施/组别	治疗方案	试验状态	结果
过继性T细胞治疗	N/A	NCT01585428	II	氟达拉滨，环磷酰胺，Young TIL，阿地白介素	二线	已完成	ORR: 18%（非宫颈癌）
	N/A	NCT03083873	II	氟达拉滨，环磷酰胺，冷冻保存/非冷冻保存TIL，阿地白介素	二线	活跃	结果待定
	N/A	NCT02421640	II	顺铂，RT，TIL/顺铂，RT	一线	未知	结果待定

CTLA-4：细胞毒性T淋巴细胞相关抗原4；ICOS：诱导性共刺激分子；LAG-3：淋巴细胞活化基因3；TIGIT：T细胞免疫球蛋白及免疫受体酪氨酸基抑制基序；IDO1：吲哚胺-2,3-双加氧酶1；NKG2A：NK组2成员A；VISTA：T细胞活化的V结构域Ig抑制因子；SoC：标准治疗；RT：放射治疗；ORR：总缓解率；DCR：疾病控制率；TIL：肿瘤浸润性淋巴细胞；N/A：不适用

Th2 分化以及效应性 CD4+ T 细胞分化中具有重要作用[19]。在黑色素瘤小鼠模型中，ICOS 主要由 Th1 细胞表达，并可与抗 CTLA-4 治疗发生协同作用，共同促进肿瘤清除[20]。此外，研究显示，在小鼠中，抑制 PD-1/PD-L1 通路可通过在生发中心激活 ERK 信号通路增强 CD4+ T 细胞中 ICOS 的表达，从而提高体液免疫[21]；抑制 PD-1/PD-L1 通路还能提高肿瘤浸润性淋巴细胞（TIL）中 ICOS 的水平[22]。这些发现为靶向 ICOS 和联合 PD-1/PD-L1 的联合治疗提供了依据。

Ⅲ期 INDUCE-3 试验（NCT04128696）和 INDUCE-4 试验（NCT04428333）在 PD-L1 阳性（CPS ≥ 1）的 R/M HNC 患者中评估了 ICOS 激动性单抗 feladilimab 在一线治疗中的疗效，该试验比较了 feladilimab 联合帕博利珠单抗、安慰剂加帕博利珠单抗，以及铂类化疗联合 5-FU 的疗效。在基于前 140 例患者（随访时间 ≥ 22 周）的计划中期分析中，feladilimab 联合帕博利珠单抗组的总缓解率（ORR）为 18.6%（13/70，95%CI：10.3%~29.7%；包括 2 例完全缓解（complete response，CR）和 11 例部分缓解（partial response，PR），而安慰剂加帕博利珠单抗组的 ORR 为 30%（21/70，95%CI：19.6%~42.1%；包括 2 例 CR 和 19 例 PR）。在审查 INDUCE-3 试验数据后，独立数据监测委员会（Independent Data Monitoring Committee，IDMC）建议停止该研究，因为其未能达到预设的继续试验标准。另一种 ICOS 激动剂 BMS-986226 在晚期实体瘤中的疗效目前正在 Ⅰ/Ⅱ期临床试验（NCT03251924）中被评估，涉及单药治疗以及与纳武利尤单抗或伊匹木单抗联合治疗。

4 淋巴细胞活化基因 3（LAG-3, CD223）

淋巴细胞活化基因 3（LAG-3）是免疫球蛋白超家族的跨膜蛋白，也被认为是肿瘤免疫逃逸的促进因子。LAG-3 的编码基因最早由 Triebel 等在 30 多年前发现[23]，其基因组结构与 CD4 密切相关[24]。LAG-3 主要在调节性 T 细胞（Treg）中表达，并与 IL-10 的产生增加相关。它也在活化的 T 细胞、B 细胞、树突细胞和 NK 细胞中表达，并可通过抑制 T 细胞的增殖和活性发挥作用[25]。已确定的 LAG-3 配体包括主要组织相容性复合体Ⅱ（MHCⅡ）、肝和淋巴结窦状内皮细胞C型凝集素（liver and lymph node sinusoidal endothelial cell C-type lectin, LSECtin）、半乳凝素3（GAL-3）和纤维蛋白原样蛋白1（fibrinogen-like protein 1, FGL-1）[26]。LAG-3与MHCⅡ之间的亲和力高于MHCⅡ与CD4受体之间的亲和力，从而导致CD4+ T细胞失活[27]。LAG-3也可通过上调免疫受体酪氨酸活化基序（immunoreceptor tyrosine-based activation motif, ITAM）信号抑制树突细胞功能[28]。此外，研究表明LAG-3还可通过TCR依赖性机制抑制肿瘤内和外周CD8+ T细胞的效应功能，这一机制可能由IL-6和IL-8水平升高诱导[29]。在HNC中，肿瘤浸润性淋巴细胞中LAG-3的高表达与更高的病理分级、肿瘤分期及淋巴结阳性相关。在人类HNC的小鼠模型中，LAG-3被证明是独立的不良预后指标，而通过靶向性单抗阻断LAG-3可导致肿瘤缩小[30]。

在B16黑色素瘤、MC38结肠腺癌和Sa1N纤维肉瘤小鼠模型中，LAG-3通路的抑制能与PD-1抑制剂产生协同作用，从而使抗肿瘤T细胞功能增强。联合抑制这两个免疫检查点导致肿瘤缩小，其机制可能是升高肿瘤浸润的IFN-γ+CD4+ T细胞、IFN-γ+CD8+ T细胞以及TNF-α+CD4+ T细胞和TNF-α+CD8+ T细胞水平[31]。

目前有两项试验正在评估抗LAG-3药物relatlimab与抗PD-1药物纳武利尤单抗联合治疗的安全性和有效性。第一项临床试验（NCT04080804）在新辅助治疗中比较了纳武利尤单抗联合relatlimab、纳武利尤单抗联合伊匹木单抗、纳武利尤单抗单药治疗。第二项临床试验（NCT04326257）在PD-1/PD-L1抑制剂单药治疗失败的患者中评估纳武利尤单抗联合relatlimab或纳武利尤单抗联合伊匹木单抗。

另外一项TACTI-002试验（NCT03625323）评估了eftilagimod alpha（一种可溶性LAG-3融合蛋白）联合帕博利珠单抗作为免疫检查点抑制剂初治的R/M HNC患者二线治疗的疗效，初步结果显示总缓解率（ORR）为39%，疾病控制率（disease control rate, DCR）为50%[32]。同样的联合方案在不可切除或转移性黑色素瘤的研究中也取得了积极结果。根据Ⅰ期TACTI-mel试验（NCT02676869）数据，eftilagimod alpha联合帕博利珠单抗在帕博利珠单抗耐药患者中的ORR为33%，而在PD-1抑制剂初治的患者中ORR达50%[33]。

5 T细胞免疫球蛋白及免疫受体酪氨酸基抑制基序（TIGIT）

T细胞免疫球蛋白及免疫受体酪氨酸基抑制性基序（T cell immunoglobulin and immunoreceptor tyrosine-based inhibitory motif, TIGIT）是一种共抑制受体分子，属于脊髓灰质炎病毒受体（poliovirus receptor, PVR）家族的免疫球蛋白，主要表达于淋巴细胞中，包括效应 CD4+ 和 CD8+ T 细胞、调节性 CD4+ T 细胞（Treg）、滤泡辅助 T 细胞和 NK 细胞[34]。脊髓灰质炎病毒受体（PVR/Nectin-like-5/CD155）是 TIGIT 的高亲和力配体（PVRL2/Nectin-2/CD112 和 PVRL3/Nectin-3/CD113 也可与 TIGIT 结合，但亲和力较低），其在内皮细胞、成纤维细胞、树突细胞和肿瘤细胞中高表达[35]。

临床前研究表明，TIGIT 表达的 NK 细胞与表达 CD155 的髓源性抑制细胞（MDSC）相互作用后，其抗肿瘤细胞毒性显著降低，而这种作用可以通过阻断 TIGIT 或活性氧逆转[36]。此外，TIGIT 的表达是一种高度活化的免疫抑制型 Treg 亚群的特征，这一亚群在小鼠肿瘤模型中与 TIM-3 协同作用，促进肿瘤免疫逃逸[37]。在黑色素瘤模型中，CD155 通过与 TIGIT 相互作用抑制肿瘤特异性细胞毒性 T 细胞的细胞因子释放[38]。研究还发现，TIGIT 与 PD-1 在肿瘤浸润性 CD8+ T 细胞中共表达，并在 PD-1 抑制后进一步上调。然而，同时阻断 TIGIT 和 PD-1 显著增强了肿瘤抗原特异性和肿瘤浸润性 CD8+ T 细胞的增殖和活化[39]。

在头颈部肿瘤中，Wu 等研究发现，患者样本及小鼠模型中的肿瘤浸润性 CD4+ T 细胞和 CD8+ T 细胞（TIL）中 TIGIT 表达水平升高，同时肿瘤细胞或 TIL 中 CD155 表达水平对预后具有负面影响。阻断 TIGIT 能够显著减缓 HNC 小鼠模型中的肿瘤生长，可能与治疗后 IL-2、TNF-α 和 IFN-γ 表达增加的 CD8+ T 细胞以及 IL-2 表达增加的 CD4+ T 细胞水平相关。此外，TIGIT 抑制还导致 Treg 和 MDSC 活性的降低[40]。TIGIT 抑制剂 tiragolumab 目前正在随机 II 期 SKYSCRAPER-09 试验（NCT04665843）中进行研究，该试验在 PD-L1 阳性的 R/M HNC 患者中比较了作为一线治疗的 tiragolumab 联合 PD-L1 抑制剂 atezolizumab 与 atezolizumab 加安慰剂的疗效。

6　T 细胞免疫球蛋白黏蛋白 3（TIM-3）

TIM-3 是细胞免疫球蛋白黏蛋白（T cell immunoglobulin mucin, TIM）家族的一个成员，主要表达于 CD4+ Th1 细胞、Treg、CD8+ T 细胞、树突细胞、NK 细胞、单核细胞、肥大细胞及某些肿瘤细胞，是另一种参与肿瘤免疫耐受的抑制分子。TIM-3 与其主要配体半乳凝素 9（GAL-9）结合后，已被证实可抑制 Th1 和 Th17 细胞的增殖，诱导 Th1 细胞凋亡、CD8+ T 细胞失活以及 MDSC 扩增。Liu 等研究表明，在 HNC 小鼠模型中，可以升高浸润性效应 T 细胞（effector T cell, Teff）的水平，激活 CXCL1，从而减少 MDSC，从而抑制肿瘤生长[41]。TIM-3 抑制还能刺激 CD8+ T 细胞的 IFN-γ 分泌，并降低 Treg 密度[42]。此外，在 HNC 小鼠模型中，TIM-3 抑制被证明能够增强放疗和 PD-L1 抑制剂联合治疗的疗效。尽管放疗或 PD-L1 抑制后 CD8+ T 细胞和 Treg 的 TIM-3 表达显著增加，但随后的 TIM-3 抑制能够恢复细胞毒性，减少 Treg 群体并延长生存期[43]。抗 TIM-3 药物 sabatolimab（MBG453）、cobolimab（TSR-022）和 LY3321367 目前正在多个早期临床试验（NCT026082268、NCT02817633 和 NCT03099109）中进行研究，涉及单药治疗或与抗 PD-1/PD-L1 药物联合治疗多种晚期肿瘤。

7　吲哚胺 -2,3- 双加氧酶 1（IDO1）

吲哚胺 -2,3- 双加氧酶 1（indoleamine-pyrrole 2,3-dioxygenase 1, IDO1）是一种重要的限速酶，在色氨酸（Trp）代谢为犬尿氨酸（kynurenine）及其终产物的过程中发挥核心作用。它通过多种机制参与免疫抑制，包括 Trp 耗竭引发的 T 细胞无能现象，该过程涉及 GCN2 和 mTOR 信号通路。此外，犬尿氨酸及其代谢产物与效应 T 细胞的细胞周期停滞和凋亡相关，同时还可促进调节性 T 细胞的分化。在小鼠肿瘤模型中，IDO1 抑制被认为还与一种独立于其酶活性的免疫调节机制相关，该机制涉及 IDO1 内在的免疫受体酪氨酸基抑制基序（immunoreceptor tyrosine-based inhibitory motif，ITIM）[44]。在局部晚期 HNC 中，研究发现放化疗后 IDO1 和 PD-L1 表达水平的降低与患者无进展生存期的改善密切相关[45]。此外，在 HPV 相关 HNC 的体外研究中，联合阻断 PD-1 和 IDO1 被证明可以恢复 CD8+ T 细胞的细胞毒性功能[46]。HNC 中 IDO1 抑制剂的临床研究重点关注其与 PD-1/PD-L1 抑制剂的联合应用，已显示出一定的治疗潜力。在 ECHO-202/KEYNOTE-037 试验中，IDO1 抑制剂 epacadostat 联合帕博利珠单抗治疗既往接受过治疗的 HNC 患者，结果显示总缓解率为 34%，疾病控制率为 62%，治疗的安全性与帕博利珠单抗单药治疗相当[47]。ECHO-304/KEYNOTE-669 试验是一项Ⅲ期随机开放标签研究，在 R/M HNC 患者的一线治疗中评估了以下方案：epacadostat 联合帕博利珠单抗、帕博利珠单抗单药治疗、EXTREME 方案，目前该研究正在进行中[48]。ECHO-204 试验评估了 epacadostat 联合纳武利尤单抗的疗效，初步结果显示 R/M HNC 患者的疾病控制率达到 70%[49]。ECHO-203 试验显示 epacadostat 联合度伐利尤单抗在多种恶性肿瘤中具有良好的安全性，HNC 患者的Ⅱ期扩展队列结果尚未公布[50]。此外，还有多个关于头颈部肿瘤中应用 IDO1 抑制剂的研究正在进行中。IDO1 抑制剂 linrodostat（BMS986205）联合纳武利尤单抗正在一项Ⅱ期"治疗机会窗口"试验（NCT03854032）中被评估，用于术前治疗Ⅱ~Ⅳ期 HNC 患者。Ⅲ期 CHECKMATE 9NA/ECHO-310 试验（NCT03342352）在 HNC 患者中评估了纳武利尤单抗加 epacadostat 加化疗的联合方案与 EXTREME 方案的疗效，但由于某些原因，该研究已提前终止。

8　糖皮质激素诱导的 TNFR 相关基因（GITR）

糖皮质激素诱导的 TNFR 相关基因（glucocorticoid-induced TNFR family-related gene，GITR）是肿瘤坏死因子受体超家族（tumor necrosis factor receptor superfamily，TNFRSF）的一个成员，主要表达于活化的调节性 T 细胞（Treg），同时也存在于效应 T 细胞、NK 细胞、树突细胞和巨噬细胞表面。GITR 与其配体 GITRL 结合后被激活，GITRL 主要表达在抗原呈递细胞（APC）和内皮细胞表面，激活后可诱导多种促炎症反应[51]。

GITR 的共刺激作用机制已经通过多项研究得以阐明。在临床前模型中，GITR 被证明可以通过上调 Bcl-XL 抑制 T 细胞凋亡，增强外周 T 细胞产生 IL-2 和 IFN-γ。此外，GITR 还可通过 T 细胞受体（TCR）依赖的方式增强 CD8+ T 细胞的细胞毒性。GITR 对于 Treg 具有双重作用：起初可抑制 Treg 的免疫抑制功能，随后因 CD4+ T 细胞产生高水平的 IL-10 而促进 Th2 和 Treg 的分化和扩增。在肿瘤环境中，GITR 激活能够通过抑制 Treg 介导的免疫抑制作用增强 CD8+ 和 CD4+ 效应 T 细胞的活性[52]。

在小鼠肿瘤模型中，应用 GITR 激动性单抗 DTA-1 可以诱导多种肿瘤的缩小，为其在临床应用中的研究奠定了基础[52]。AMG 228（IgG1 型单抗）是一种 GITR 激动剂，Ⅰ期临床试验（NCT02437916）评估了其在晚期非小细胞肺癌、黑色素瘤、结肠癌和头颈部肿瘤中的安全性、药代动力学、药效学及最大耐受剂量（maximum tolerated dose，MTD）。结果显示，该药物具有良好的耐受性，并未达到 MTD，但未观察到显著的 T 细胞激活或抗肿瘤效应[53]。

9　CD94/NKG2A

NKG2A 即 NK 组 2 成员 A（NK group 2 member A）。CD94/NKG2A 是 NK 细胞和 CD8+ T 细胞表面发现的异二聚体形的抑制性受体。CD94/NKG2A 通过与肿瘤细胞表达的 HLA-E 结合引发 TCR 依赖的免疫抑制作用，从而降低 NK 细胞和 CD8+ T 细胞的细胞毒性，包括抗体依赖性细胞介导的细胞毒性[54]。研究表明，阻断 NKG2A 能够增强 T 细胞和 NK 细胞的活性，从而促进抗肿瘤反应[55]。在头颈部肿瘤中，CD8+ 肿瘤浸润性淋巴细胞（TIL）中 NKG2A 表达增加以及肿瘤细胞中

HLA-E 表达增加，为靶向该通路的治疗提供了理论依据[56]。

monalizumab 是第一个用于头颈部肿瘤患者的抗 NKG2A 药物。UPSTREAM 研究（NCT03088059）是一项基于生物标志物的多队列研究，评估了多种药物及其组合在铂类治疗失败的头颈部肿瘤患者中的疗效；然而 monalizumab 治疗组未达到主要研究终点，因为未观察到客观缓解；目前在接受过 PD-1/PD-L1 抗体治疗的患者中，将 monalizumab 联合度伐利尤单抗与标准治疗方案进行比较的研究正在进行[57]。monalizumab 在头颈部肿瘤中的应用研究还包括一项在既往既往接受过治疗的 R/M HNC 患者中进行的Ⅰ/Ⅱ期临床试验（NCT02643550），该试验评估了 monalizumab 联合西妥昔单抗的疗效，结果显示：ORR 为 27.5%，其中包括 1 例完全缓解（2.5%）和 10 例部分缓解（25%）；24 周的疾病控制率为 35%，中位无进展生存期和总生存期分别为 5.0 个月和 10.3 个月；在 17 例既往接受 PD-1/PD-L1 抗体治疗的患者中，有 3 例患者（18%）获得缓解[58]。INTERLINK-1 试验（NCT04590963）是一项正在进行的Ⅲ期研究，在铂类耐药并接受过 PD-1/PD-L1 抗体治疗的 R/M HNC 患者中评估 monalizumab 联合西妥昔单抗与安慰剂联合西妥昔单抗的疗效。还有一项 Ib/Ⅱ期研究（NCT02331875）在 HNC 患者中评估 monalizumab 单药作为新辅助治疗的疗效，但该试验因缺乏疗效而提前终止。

10　OX40 受体（OX40R, CD134）

OX40 受体是肿瘤坏死因子受体（tumor necrosis factor receptor, TNFRTNFR）家族的成员，是一种共刺激性Ⅰ类跨膜糖蛋白，主要表达于活化的 CD4+ T 细胞表面。OX40 与其配体 OX40L 结合后，能够上调抗凋亡因子，逆转免疫抑制状态，并增强效应 T 细胞的功能。此外，应用 OX40 激动性单抗已被证明能够耗竭肿瘤微环境中的调节性 T 细胞，并降低其 IL-10 的分泌水平，从而促进树突细胞的扩增并增强抗肿瘤细胞毒性[59]。

MEDI6469 试验（NCT02274155）和 MEDI0562 试验（NCT03336606）是两项针对头颈部肿瘤的Ⅰ期研究，评估了 OX40 激动性单抗单药作为新辅助治疗的安全性及潜在治疗效果。MEDI6469 试验结果显示药物耐受性良好，并且在治疗后手术标本中观察到免疫原性增强[60]。此外，OX40 激动剂 PF-04518600 联合 PD-L1 抗体阿维鲁单抗（avelumab）正在ⅠB/Ⅱ期 JAVELIN Medley 研究（NCT02554812）中被评估，该研究涵盖了头颈部肿瘤及其他晚期恶性肿瘤。同时，OX40 靶向药物与其他免疫检查点抑制剂的联合疗法也在进行深入研究。

11 T 细胞活化 V 域免疫球蛋白抑制分子（VISTA）

T 细胞活化 V 域免疫球蛋白抑制分子（V-domain Ig suppressor of T cell activation, VISTA）是一种新型免疫检查点分子，其结构与 B7 家族其他成员差异显著。VISTA 通过抑制效应 T 细胞的激活并促进调节性 T 细胞（Treg）的增殖，在免疫调控中发挥作用。VISTA 在多种肿瘤浸润性淋巴细胞亚群中表达，包括抗原呈递细胞、初始 CD4+ T 细胞和 Treg。在肿瘤微环境中，VISTA 通过与其配体 VSIG3 结合表现出免疫抑制效应[61]。有趣的是，尽管临床前数据显示 VISTA 在几种恶性肿瘤中可以非冗余性地影响 PD-1 抑制，但在头颈部肿瘤模型中，抗 VISTA 的单克隆抗体 MIH63 会优先增强 CTLA-4 抑制剂活性，而对 PD-1 抑制剂的协同作用有限[62]。

关于 VISTA 抑制的临床研究处于非常早期的阶段。一项Ⅰ期临床试验（NCT02671955）在包括头颈部肿瘤在内的晚期肿瘤患者中评估抗 VISTA 的全人源化 IgG1 Kappa 单抗 onvatilimab 的作用，但该试验因资助方决定而提前终止。一项Ⅰ期研究（NCT02812875）评估了 CA-170（针对 PD-1/PD-L1 和 VISTA 的口服双重抑制剂）在晚期恶性肿瘤中的疗效，目前尚未报告结果[63]。另外一项正在进行的Ⅰ期试验（NCT04475523）评估抗 VISTA 的单克隆抗体 CI-8993 在晚期实体瘤中的疗效，目前正在招募患者。

12　替代策略：过继细胞疗法

免疫检查点阻断（immune checkpoint blockade, ICB）策略的成功应用为基于免疫细胞操控的其他治疗方法的发展奠定了基础，其目标是利用免疫细胞靶向肿瘤特异性靶点。过继性 T 细胞治疗被用于克服 ICB 的局限性，比如 ICB 策略需要预先存在免疫浸润，在预先缺乏免疫浸润或免疫耗竭的患者中就可应用过继性 T 细胞治疗。这一技术包括从患者的肿瘤浸润性淋巴细胞（TIL）中分离 T 细胞，随后体外扩增和选择所需的亚群细胞，并将这些细胞重新输注回患者体内。大多数临床试验采用非骨髓抑制性淋巴细胞耗竭化疗方案，在细胞输注前采用氟达拉滨和环磷酰胺处理，并在细胞输注后给予 T 细胞生长因子（如白介素 2）[64]。

目前在包括头颈部肿瘤在内的几种恶性肿瘤中过继性 T 细胞治疗处于临床评估阶段。在一项 HPV 相关实体瘤的 I 期临床试验（NCT01585428）中，11 名非宫颈癌患者中有 2 名通过非骨髓抑制性化疗（使用氟达拉滨和环磷酰胺）联合 TIL 输注和 IL-2 刺激实现部分缓解[65]。同样的治疗方案目前正在另一项针对 R/M HNC 的 II 期试验（NCT03083873）中进行评估 [66]。

13　结论

免疫检查点抑制已成为复发/转移性头颈部肿瘤的重要治疗方法，为患者提供了显著的临床益处。然而，肿瘤微环境中复杂的免疫细胞相互作用凸显了靶向其他协同或拮抗免疫调节分子的必要性，以最大化宿主的抗肿瘤免疫反应。在这一背景下，多种免疫检查点的研究推动了相关靶向药物的开发，为未来头颈部肿瘤治疗的转型奠定了基础。

原文符合伦理标准相关声明

Disclosure of Potential Conflicts of Interest　AP has received honoraria from Astrazeneca, Bayer, BMS, Genesis Pharmaceuticals, Merck, Serono, MSD Oncology, Pfizer, Rakuten

Medical, and Roche. AP has served as an advisor for Amgen, AstraZeneca, Bristol-Myers Squibb, eTheRNA immunotherapies, MSD Oncology, Pfizer, and Rakuten Medical. AP has received research funding by Amgen, Boehringer Ingelheim, Bristol-Myers Squibb, Demo Pharmaceutical, Kura Oncology, Pfizer, Pharmathen, and Roche and has received travel, accommodations, and expenses funding by Bristol-Myers Squibb, Ipsen, MSD Oncology, and Roche. Other authors have no potential conflicts of interest.

参考文献

1. Gupta B, Johnson NW, Kumar N (2016) Global epidemiology of head and neck cancers: a continuing challenge. Oncology 91(1):13-23. https://doi.org/10.1159/000446117
2. Sung H, Ferlay J, Siegel RL et al (2021) Global cancer statistics 2020: GLOBOCAN estimates of incidence and mortality worldwide for 36 cancers in 185 countries. CA Cancer J Clin 71(3):209-249. https://doi.org/10.3322/caac.21660
3. de Martel C, Plummer M, Vignat J et al (2017) Worldwide burden of cancer attributable to HPV by site, country and HPV type. Int J Cancer 141(4):664-670. https://doi.org/10.1002/ijc.30716
4. Rampias T, Sasaki C, Weinberger P et al (2009) E6 and e7 gene silencing and transformed phenotype of human papillomavirus 16-positive oropharyngeal cancer cells. J Natl Cancer Inst 101(6):412-423. https://doi.org/10.1093/jnci/djp017
5. Chung CH, Guthrie VB, Masica DL et al (2015) Genomic alterations in head and neck squamous cell carcinoma determined by cancer gene-targeted sequencing. Ann Oncol 26(6):1216-1223. https://doi.org/10.1093/annonc/mdv109
6. South AP, den Breems NY, Richa T et al (2019) Mutation signature analysis identifies increased mutation caused by tobacco smoke associated DNA adducts in larynx squamous cell carcinoma compared with oral cavity and oropharynx. Sci Rep 9(1):19256. https://doi.org/10.1038/s41598-019-55352-y
7. Koo BS, Lim YC, Lee JS et al (2006) Recurrence and salvage treatment of squamous cell carcinoma of the oral cavity. Oral Oncol 42(8):789-794. https://doi.org/10.1016/j.oraloncology.2005.11.016
8. Ang KK, Harris J, Wheeler R et al (2010) Human papillomavirus and survival of patients with oropharyngeal cancer. N Engl J Med 363(1):24-35. https://doi.org/10.1056/NEJMoa0912217
9. Machiels JP, Rene Leemans C, Golusinski W et al (2020) Squamous cell carcinoma of the oral cavity, larynx, oropharynx and hypopharynx: EHNS-ESMO-ESTRO clinical practice guidelines for diagnosis, treatment and follow-up. Ann Oncol 31(11):1462-1475. https://doi.org/10.1016/j.annonc.2020.07.011
10. Le X, Ferrarotto R, Wise-Draper T et al (2020) Evolving role of immunotherapy in recurrent metastatic head and neck cancer. J Natl Compr Cancer Netw 18(7):899-906. https://doi.org/10.6004/jnccn.2020.7590
11. Linsley PS, Bradshaw J, Greene J et al (1996) Intracellular trafficking of CTLA-4 and focal localization towards sites of TCR engagement. Immunity 4(6):535-543. https://doi.org/10.1016/s1074-7613(00)80480-x
12. Rowshanravan B, Halliday N, Sansom DM (2018) CTLA-4: a moving target in immunotherapy. Blood 131(1):58-67. https://doi.org/10.1182/blood-2017-06-741033
13. Yu GT, Bu LL, Zhao YY et al (2016) CTLA4 blockade reduces immature myeloid cells in head

and neck squamous cell carcinoma. Oncoimmunology 5(6):e1151594. https://doi.org/10.1080/2162402X.2016.1151594
14. Wang Z, Wu VH, Allevato MM et al (2019) Syngeneic animal models of tobacco-associated oral cancer reveal the activity of in situ anti-CTLA-4. Nat Commun 10(1):5546. https://doi.org/10.1038/s41467-019-13471-0
15. Lipson EJ, Drake CG (2011) Ipilimumab: an anti-CTLA-4 antibody for metastatic melanoma. Clin Cancer Res 17(22):6958-6962. https://doi.org/10.1158/1078-0432. CCR-11-1595
16. Siu LL, Even C, Mesia R et al (2019) Safety and efficacy of durvalumab with or without tremelimumab in patients with PD-L1-low/negative recurrent or metastatic HNSCC: the phase 2 CONDOR randomized clinical trial. JAMA Oncol 5(2):195-203. https://doi.org/10.1001/jamaoncol.2018.4628
17. Ferris RL, Haddad R, Even C et al (2020) Durvalumab with or without tremelimumab in patients with recurrent or metastatic head and neck squamous cell carcinoma: EAGLE, a randomized, open-label phase III study. Ann Oncol 31(7):942-950. https://doi.org/10.1016/j.annonc.2020.04.001
18. Argiris A, Gillison M, Ferris RL et al (2016) A randomized, open-label, phase 3 study of nivolumab in combination with ipilimumab vs extreme regimen (cetuximab + cisplatin/carboplatin + fluorouracil) as first-line therapy in patients with recurrent or metastatic squamous cell carcinoma of the head and neck-CheckMate 651. Ann Oncol 27:vi350. https://doi.org/10.1093/annonc/mdw376.68
19. Wikenheiser DJ, Stumhofer JS (2016) ICOS co-stimulation: friend or foe? Front Immunol. https://doi.org/10.3389/fimmu.2016.00304
20. Fu T, He Q, Sharma P (2011) The ICOS/ICOSL pathway is required for optimal antitumor responses mediated by anti-CTLA-4 therapy. Cancer Res 71(16):5445-5454. https://doi.org/10.1158/0008-5472. CAN-11-1138
21. Zhang M, Xia L, Yang Y et al (2019) PD-1 blockade augments humoral immunity through ICOS-mediated CD4(+) T cell instruction. Int Immunopharmacol 66:127-138. https://doi.org/10.1016/j.intimp.2018.10.045
22. Beyrend G, van der Gracht E, Yilmaz A et al (2019) PD-L1 blockade engages tumor-infiltrating lymphocytes to co-express targetable activating and inhibitory receptors. J Immunother Cancer 7(1):217. https://doi.org/10.1186/s40425-019-0700-3
23. Triebel F, Jitsukawa S, Baixeras E et al (1990) LAG-3, a novel lymphocyte activation gene closely related to CD4. J Exp Med 171(5):1393-1405. https://doi.org/10.1084/jem.171.5.1393
24. Bruniquel D, Borie N, Triebel F (1997) Genomic organization of the human LAG-3/CD4 locus. Immunogenetics 47(1):96-98. https://doi.org/10.1007/s002510050332
25. Huard B, Tournier M, Hercend T et al (1994) Lymphocyte-activation gene 3/major histocompatibility complex class II interaction modulates the antigenic response of CD4+ T lymphocytes. Eur J Immunol 24(12):3216-3221. https://doi.org/10.1002/eji.1830241246
26. Maruhashi T, Sugiura D, Okazaki IM et al (2020) LAG-3: from molecular functions to clinical applications. J Immunother Cancer. https://doi.org/10.1136/jitc-2020-001014
27. Workman CJ, Dugger KJ, Vignali DA (2002) Cutting edge: molecular analysis of the negative regulatory function of lymphocyte activation gene-3. J Immunol 169(10):5392-5395. https://doi.org/10.4049/jimmunol.169.10.5392
28. Liang B, Workman C, Lee J et al (2008) Regulatory T cells inhibit dendritic cells by lymphocyte

activation gene-3 engagement of MHC class II. J Immunol 180(9):5916-5926. https://doi.org/10.4049/jimmunol.180.9.5916
29. Somasundaram A, Cillo AR, Lampenfeld C et al (2020) Systemic immune dysfunction in cancer patients driven by IL6 and IL8 induction of an inhibitory receptor module in peripheral CD8+T cells. bioRxiv. https://doi.org/10.1101/2020.05.06.081471
30. Deng WW, Mao L, Yu GT et al (2016) LAG-3 confers poor prognosis and its blockade reshapes antitumor response in head and neck squamous cell carcinoma. Oncoimmunology 5(11):e1239005. https://doi.org/10.1080/2162402X.2016.1239005
31. Woo SR, Turnis ME, Goldberg MV et al (2012) Immune inhibitory molecules LAG-3 and PD-1 synergistically regulate T-cell function to promote tumoral immune escape. Cancer Res 72(4):917-927. https://doi.org/10.1158/0008-5472.CAN-11-1620
32. Forster M, Felip E, Doger B et al (2020) 927P Initial results from a phase II study (TACTI-002) of eftilagimod alpha (soluble LAG-3 protein) and pembrolizumab as 2nd line treatment for PD-L1 unselected metastatic head and neck cancer patients. Ann Oncol 31:S667. https://doi.org/10.1016/annonc/annonc277
33. Atkinson V, Khattak A, Haydon A et al (2020) Eftilagimod alpha, a soluble lymphocyte activation gene-3 (LAG-3) protein plus pembrolizumab in patients with metastatic melanoma. J Immunother Cancer. https://doi.org/10.1136/jitc-2020-001681
34. Yu X, Harden K, Gonzalez LC et al (2009) The surface protein TIGIT suppresses T cell activation by promoting the generation of mature immunoregulatory dendritic cells. Nat Immunol 10(1):48-57. https://doi.org/10.1038/ni.1674
35. Manieri NA, Chiang EY, Grogan JL (2017) TIGIT: a key inhibitor of the cancer immunity cycle. Trends Immunol 38(1):20-28. https://doi.org/10.1016/j.it.2016.10.002
36. Sarhan D, Cichocki F, Zhang B et al (2016) Adaptive NK cells with low TIGIT expression are inherently resistant to myeloid-derived suppressor cells. Cancer Res 76(19):5696-5706. https://doi.org/10.1158/0008-5472.CAN-16-0839
37. Kurtulus S, Sakuishi K, Ngiow SF et al (2015) TIGIT predominantly regulates the immune response via regulatory T cells. J Clin Invest 125(11):4053-4062. https://doi.org/10.1172/JCI81187
38. Inozume T, Yaguchi T, Furuta J et al (2016) Melanoma cells control antimelanoma CTL responses via interaction between TIGIT and CD155 in the effector phase. J Invest Dermatol 136(1):255-263. https://doi.org/10.1038/JID.2015.404
39. Chauvin JM, Pagliano O, Fourcade J et al (2015) TIGIT and PD-1 impair tumor antigen-specific CD8(+) T cells in melanoma patients. J Clin Invest 125(5):2046-2058. https://doi.org/10.1172/JCI80445
40. Wu L, Mao L, Liu JF et al (2019) Blockade of TIGIT/CD155 signaling reverses T-cell exhaustion and enhances antitumor capability in head and neck squamous cell carcinoma. Cancer Immunol Res 7(10):1700-1713. https://doi.org/10.1158/2326-6066.CIR-18-0725
41. Liu J-F, Ma S-R, Mao L et al (2017) T-cell immunoglobulin mucin 3 blockade drives an antitumor immune response in head and neck cancer. Mol Oncol 11(2):235-247. https://doi.org/10.1002/1878-0261.12029
42. Liu JF, Wu L, Yang LL et al (2018) Blockade of TIM3 relieves immunosuppression through reducing regulatory T cells in head and neck cancer. J Exp Clin Cancer Res 37(1):44. https://doi.org/10.1186/s13046-018-0713-7

43. Oweida A, Hararah MK, Phan A et al (2018) Resistance to radiotherapy and PD-L1 blockade is mediated by TIM-3 upregulation and regulatory T-cell infiltration. Clin Cancer Res 24(21):5368-5380. https://doi.org/10.1158/1078-0432. CCR-18-1038
44. Zhai L, Ladomersky E, Lenzen A et al (2018) IDO1 in cancer: a Gemini of immune checkpoints. Cell Mol Immunol 15(5):447-457. https://doi.org/10.1038/cmi.2017.143
45. Economopoulou P, Kladi-Skandali A et al (2020) Prognostic impact of indoleamine 2,3-dioxygenase 1 (IDO1) mRNA expression on circulating tumour cells of patients with head and neck squamous cell carcinoma. ESMO Open 5(3):e000646. https://doi.org/10.1136/esmoopen-2019-000646
46. Krishna S, Ulrich P, Wilson E et al (2018) Human papilloma virus specific immunogenicity and dysfunction of CD8(+) T cells in head and neck cancer. Cancer Res 78(21):6159-6170. https://doi.org/10.1158/0008-5472. CAN-18-0163
47. Hamid O, Bauer TM, Spira AI et al (2017) Epacadostat plus pembrolizumab in patients with SCCHN: preliminary phase I/II results from ECHO-202/KEYNOTE-037. J Clin Oncol 35(15_Suppl):6010. https://doi.org/10.1200/JCO.2017.35.15_suppl.6010
48. Cohen EEW, Rischin D, Pfister DG et al (2018) A phase 3, randomized, open-label study of epacadostat plus pembrolizumab, pembrolizumab monotherapy, and the EXTREME regimen as first-line treatment for recurrent/metastatic head and neck squamous cell carcinoma (R/M SCCHN): ECHO-304/KEYNOTE-669. J Clin Oncol 36(15_Suppl):TPS6090. https://doi.org/10.1200/JCO.2018.36.15_suppl.TPS6090
49. Perez RP, Riese MJ, Lewis KD et al (2017) Epacadostat plus nivolumab in patients with advanced solid tumors: preliminary phase I/II results of ECHO-204. J Clin Oncol 35(15_Suppl):3003. https://doi.org/10.1200/JCO.2017.35.15_suppl.3003
50. Naing A, Powderly JD, Falchook G et al (2018) Abstract CT177—Epacadostat plus durvalumab in patients with advanced solid tumors: preliminary results of the ongoing, open-label, phase I/II ECHO-203 study. AACR annual meeting 2018 session CTMS03—biomarkers in immuno-oncology. Cancer Res. https://doi.org/10.1158/1538-7445. AM2018-CT177
51. Nocentini G, Riccardi C (2009) GITR: a modulator of immune response and inflammation. Adv Exp Med Biol 647:156-173. https://doi.org/10.1007/978-0-387-89520-8_11
52. Buzzatti G, Dellepiane C, Del Mastro L (2020) New emerging targets in cancer immunotherapy: the role of GITR. ESMO Open 4(Suppl 3):e000738. https://doi.org/10.1136/esmoopen-2020-000738
53. Tran B, Carvajal RD, Marabelle A et al (2018) Dose escalation results from a first-in-human, phase 1 study of glucocorticoid-induced TNF receptor-related protein agonist AMG 228 in patients with advanced solid tumors. J Immunother Cancer 6(1):93. https://doi.org/10.1186/s40425-018-0407-x
54. Creelan BC, Antonia SJ (2019) The NKG2A immune checkpoint—a new direction in cancer immunotherapy. Nat Rev Clin Oncol 16(5):277-278. https://doi.org/10.1038/s41571-019-0182-8
55. André P, Denis C, Soulas C et al (2018) Anti-NKG2A mAb is a checkpoint inhibitor that promotes anti-tumor immunity by unleashing both T and NK cells. Cell 175(7):1731-1743.e1713. https://doi.org/10.1016/j.cell.2018.10.014
56. Charap AJ, Enokida T, Brody R et al (2020) Landscape of natural killer cell activity in head and neck squamous cell carcinoma. J Immunother Cancer. https://doi.org/10.1136/jitc-2020-001523
57. Galot R, Le Tourneau C, Saada-Bouzid E et al (2019) A phase II study of monalizumab in patients

with recurrent/metastatic (RM) squamous cell carcinoma of the head and neck (SCCHN): results of the I1 cohort of the EORTC-HNCG-1559 trial (UPSTREAM). Ann Oncol 30:v449-v450. https://doi.org/10.1093/annonc/mdz252.001
58. Fayette J, Lefebvre G, Posner MR et al (2018) Results of a phase II study evaluating monalizumab in combination with cetuximab in previously treated recurrent or metastatic squamous cell carcinoma of the head and neck (R/M SCCHN). Ann Oncol 29(Suppl_8):viii372-viii399. https://doi.org/10.1093/annonc/mdy287
59. Alves Costa Silva C, Facchinetti F, Routy B et al (2020) New pathways in immune stimulation: targeting OX40. ESMO Open 5(1):e000573. https://doi.org/10.1136/esmoopen-2019-000573
60. Bell RB, Duhen R, Leidner RS et al (2018) Neoadjuvant anti-OX40 (MEDI6469) prior to surgery in head and neck squamous cell carcinoma. J Clin Oncol 36(15_Suppl):6011. https://doi.org/10.1200/JCO.2018.36.15_suppl.6011
61. ElTanbouly MA, Croteau W, Noelle RJ et al (2019) VISTA: a novel immunotherapy target for normalizing innate and adaptive immunity. Semin Immunol 42:101308. https://doi.org/10.1016/j.smim.2019.101308
62. Kondo Y, Ohno T, Nishii N et al (2016) Differential contribution of three immune checkpoint (VISTA, CTLA-4, PD-1) pathways to antitumor responses against squamous cell carcinoma. Oral Oncol 57:54-60. https://doi.org/10.1016/j.oraloncology.2016.04.005
63. Lee JJ, Powderly JD, Patel MR et al (2017) Phase 1 trial of CA-170, a novel oral small molecule dual inhibitor of immune checkpoints PD-1 and VISTA, in patients (pts) with advanced solid tumor or lymphomas. J Clin Oncol 36(15_Suppl):TPS3099. https://doi.org/10.1200/JCO.2017.35.15_suppl.TPS3099
64. Qureshi HA, Lee SM (2019) Immunotherapy approaches beyond PD-1 inhibition: the future of cellular therapy for head and neck squamous cell carcinoma. Curr Treat Options in Oncol 20(4):31. https://doi.org/10.1007/s11864-019-0630-9
65. Stevanovic S, Helman SR, Wunderlich JR et al (2018) Treatment of metastatic human papillomavirus-associated epithelial cancers with adoptive transfer of tumor-infiltrating T cells. J Clin Oncol 36(15_Suppl):3004. https://doi.org/10.1200/JCO.2018.36.15_suppl.3004
66. Leidner RS, Sukari A, Chung CH et al (2018) A phase 2, multicenter study to evaluate the efficacy and safety of autologous tumor infiltrating lymphocytes (LN-145) for the treatment of patients with recurrent and/or metastatic squamous cell carcinoma of the head and neck (HNSCC). J Clin Oncol 36(15_Suppl):TPS6096. https://doi.org/10.1200/JCO.2018.36.15_suppl.TPS6096

第6章 免疫治疗联合放疗在头颈部肿瘤中的转化与临床研究

Translational and Clinical Approach to Combining Immunotherapy with Radiotherapy in the Treatment of Head and Neck Cancer

（Quaovi H. Sodji, Dhanya K. Nambiar, Quynh-Thu Le　著）
（韩光，袁程，徐璐，易廷庄　译）

摘要

在20世纪，免疫治疗被认为是医学史上最伟大的进步之一，为全球数百万肿瘤患者提供了一种新的治疗选择。然而，当我们开始探索其潜在价值时，我们意识到并非所有患者都能从免疫治疗中获益，原因可能是肿瘤细胞会发展出免疫逃逸机制。放疗通过免疫刺激效应有可能克服这些抵抗机制，因此放疗可以联合免疫治疗药物以增强疗效。然而，联合治疗仍有许多尚待解答的问题，包括要确定能获得最佳疗效的免疫调节剂类型、放疗剂量、分割方式、放疗与免疫治疗的顺序。本章将概述头颈部鳞状细胞癌的免疫逃逸和耐药机制，探讨目前支持放疗联合免疫治疗的相关临床前证据，以期利用现有的临床数据来阐明上述问题。

原作者信息

Quaovi H. Sodji and Dhanya K. Nambiar contributed equally with all other contributors.

Q. H. Sodji · D. K. Nambiar · Q.-T. Le (✉)
Department of Radiation Oncology, Stanford Cancer Center, Stanford University School of Medicine, Stanford, CA, USA
e-mail: Qle@stanford.edu

关键词

远隔效应·头颈部鳞状细胞癌·免疫治疗·放射治疗·立体定向消融放射治疗

1　引言

2020 年，美国有超过 65 000 例头颈部恶性肿瘤的新发病例，其中有 14 500 人死于该疾病[1]。全球有超过 83 万例头颈部恶性肿瘤的新发病例，并导致了 431 131 例患者死亡[2]。大多数（66%）患者被诊断已经是晚期，其中 10% 的患者已发生远处转移[3-4]。尽管已采用各种治疗方法，但仍有 30%~40% 的局部晚期患者会出现局部复发，20%~30% 的患者会出现远处转移，凸显了对新治疗方法的需求[5-6]。此外，除了疗效不佳外，与治疗相关的毒副作用也会对患者的生活质量产生不利影响[7]。与细胞毒性化疗药物相比，免疫治疗在减轻毒副作用的同时还能获得持久的疗效，是一种变革性的肿瘤治疗手段[7]。随着免疫治疗在黑色素瘤中取得成功，人们开始关注头颈部鳞状细胞癌（HNSCC）及其免疫微环境，因为 HNSCC 通常在肿瘤微环境（TME）中具有高度炎症反应[8]。HNSCC 表现出与免疫治疗反应相关的特征，如高水平的基因组不稳定性、突变率和癌症特异性新抗原。与其他肿瘤类型相比，HNSCC 患者的肿瘤中有更多的 T 细胞浸润。对癌症基因组图谱计划（The Cancer Genome Atlas，TCGA）的 RNA 测序数据分析显示，与十种高度免疫原性肿瘤类型相比，无论 HPV 状态如何，HNSCC 肿瘤微环境中的细胞毒性 CD8+T 细胞和自然杀伤细胞的水平均升高[9]。

正如预期的那样，TME 中 CD8+T 细数量的增加与 HNSCC 患者的生存率、无病生存期和局部控制率密切相关[10]，进一步支持了免疫治疗在 HNSCC 中的应用。KEYNOTE-012 试验、KEYNOTE-040 试验和 CHECKMATE 141 试验等具有里程碑意义的临床研究促使帕博利珠单抗和纳武利尤单抗被批准用于铂类耐药的 R/M HNSCC 患者。上述研究确立了抗 PD-1 药物作为免疫检查点抑制剂在 R/M HNSCC 患者中作为单药或与化疗联合使用，为患者提供了新的治疗选择。然而抗 PD-1 药物对局部进展期肿瘤的作用尚不明确，尤其是与放疗联合使用时，这也是本章要探讨的主题。

2　免疫检查点抑制剂的耐药机制

免疫检查点抑制剂（immune checkpoint inhibitor, ICI）的耐药可分为原发性耐药和获得性耐药，前者发生在治疗开始后从未有反应的患者；后者发生在最初有反应的患者，而后病情进展才出现耐药。耐药性可能是肿瘤细胞的内在特性，肿瘤细胞可以发展出免疫逃逸机制，也可能是肿瘤细胞通过干扰 T 细胞激活而产生的外部性因素[11]。ICI 耐药的关键机制包括肿瘤免疫原性降低、抗原呈递减弱和存在免疫抑制肿瘤微环境[12]。其他重要因素包括免疫抑制因子的分泌、免疫检查点蛋白及其各自配体的过表达、主要组织相容性复合体Ⅰ（MHCⅠ）的下调、免疫抑制细胞的浸润和扩增等。

3　放疗克服对免疫检查点抑制作用的抵抗

放疗与免疫治疗药物的联合使用已被证明可诱导远隔效应，即位于照射区域外的残余肿瘤的消退。尽管远隔效应这个术语最早由 R. H. Mole 在 1953 年提出，但首次文献描述是在 1908 年，报道了 1 例局部晚期喉癌患者接受淋巴结放疗后，原发肿瘤获得完全缓解[13]。其后出现了许多关于远隔效应的报道。然而，尽管 ICI 的出现增加了远隔效应的发生率，但这种现象仍然非常罕见，并非放疗联合免疫治疗的主导性生物学效应。随着 ICI 的最新研究进展，Steel 假说的修订版本被提出，该假说涉及放疗和免疫治疗协作增强疗效的机制，这些机制包括空间协同作用、细胞毒性增强、正常组织保护、时间调节和生物学协同作用等[14]。

3.1 放疗的免疫刺激作用

除了通过 DNA 损伤诱导肿瘤细胞死亡外，放疗还可以引起免疫原性细胞死亡（immunogenic cell death, ICD），其特征是钙调蛋白转位到细胞表面，并在细胞外环境释放 ATP 和高迁移率族蛋白 B1（high mobility group box protein 1, HMGB1）。ICD 导致免疫系统的激活和启动，因此有可能增强 ICI 的疗效。此外，通过诱导新抗原的释放，放疗还可以作为原位疫苗进一步激活免疫系统（图 6-1）[15]。通过 ICD，放疗不仅可以增强 ICI 的治疗效果，还可以通过上调 MHC I 和 NKG2D 配体（NK 细胞激活受体）来刺激免疫应答[16-17]。放疗还可以通过消耗免疫抑制细胞[18]和增加促炎细胞因子的产生来调节肿瘤微环境[19]。通过上述机制，放疗可以通过增强肿瘤免疫原性和增加抗原呈递，从而将免疫"冷"肿瘤转化为"热"肿瘤，增强 ICI 疗效。

3.2 放疗降低肿瘤负荷

放疗增强 ICI 疗效的另一个重要机制是降低肿瘤负荷[20]。尤其在寡转移病灶的情况下，SABR-COMET 试验已经证明降低肿瘤负荷对生存有益[21]。放疗对肿瘤的减灭作用不仅可以根除对免疫治疗有耐药性的肿瘤克隆，而且还可以缩小活肿瘤的体积，从而产生有效的免疫应答。

3.3 放疗对疾病的局部控制

对于转移性疾病，通过放疗来降低肿瘤负荷很重要。然而，通过对患者局部病灶的控制，放疗可以增强辅助治疗中 ICI 的效应，通过上述免疫刺激效应防止局部复发或远处转移。

3.4 免疫检查点抑制剂可减轻放疗的免疫抑制作用

尽管有证据表明放疗具有免疫刺激作用，但也有研究描述了其免疫抑制作用。放疗介导的免疫抑制主要源于照射区域内 T 细胞的直接杀伤以及促炎因子如 GM-CSF、TGF-β、IL-1α 和 IL-6 的分泌，这些因子有助于招募 MDSC、Treg 和 TAM，进而抑制 T 细胞的活化和功能。此外，在放射治疗后，CD4+ T 细胞和 CD8+ T 细胞的 PD-1 表达上调。

第 6 章 免疫治疗联合放疗在头颈部肿瘤中的转化与临床研究 103

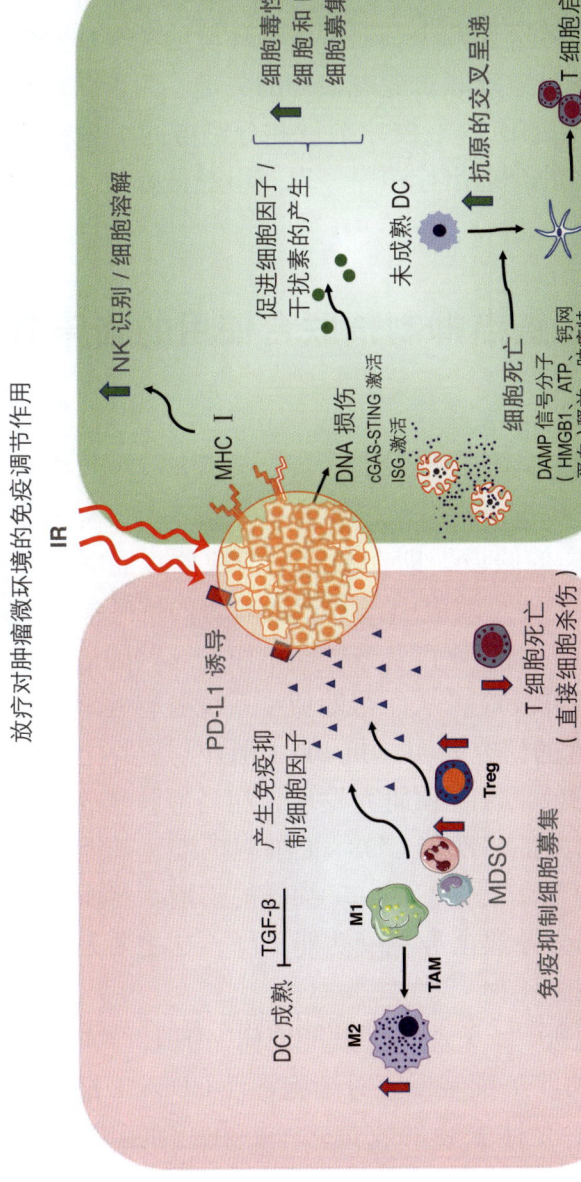

图 6-1 放疗对肿瘤及其微环境的免疫调节作用

放疗对肿瘤微环境的免疫调节作用。放疗导致免疫原性细胞死亡,其特征是向细胞外环境释放 DAMP 信号分子(钙网蛋白、ATP 和 HMGB1)[15]。DC 吸收了肿瘤细胞释放的肿瘤相关抗原后被激活并迁移到肿瘤引流淋巴结,在那里其会将抗原交叉呈递给幼稚 T 细胞。放疗还会导致恶性肿瘤细胞上的 MHC I 和 NKG2D 配体上调,并释放促炎细胞因子 [16,17,19]。放疗诱导的双链 DNA 损伤可激活 cGAS-STING-IRF3 信号转导,导致 I 型干扰素的释放。然而,放疗诱导的免疫抑制细胞因子激活会导致免疫刺激细胞(如 MDSC、Treg 和 TAM)的募集增加。放疗还会诱导巨噬细胞从 M1 型极化为 M2 型,这可能会进一步导致免疫抑制。ATP:三磷酸腺苷,DAMP:损伤相关分子模式,HMGB1:高迁移率族蛋白盒蛋白 1,MHC I:主要组织相容性复合体 I,NKG2DL:自然杀伤细胞组群 2D 配体

Sridharan 等已证明，在 HNSCC 中虽然放化疗使 CD4+ T 细胞和 CD8+ T 细胞的绝对数增加了 10%，但这些 T 细胞上的 PD-1 表达增加了 200% 以上[22]。因此，在放疗后使用 ICI 抑制 PD-1/PD-L1 通路可以防止放疗诱导的 T 细胞耗竭。

如何利用放疗的免疫刺激效应并减少其对肿瘤微环境的免疫抑制效应，对上述问题的认知与理解是放疗联合免疫治疗的关键。为了获得相应知识，我们需要进一步研究如何调整放疗剂量和分割方式，并确定放疗与选定的免疫治疗药物间的合理治疗顺序，以获得最佳疗效。

4　评估放疗和免疫检查点抑制剂联合使用的临床前研究

对小鼠肿瘤模型中进行的多项研究表明，与单一疗法或对照组相比，放疗和 PD-1/PD-L1 抑制剂联合使用可显著缩小肿瘤体积，提高生存率[23-24]。研究数据支持这样的假设，即在放疗之前或放疗同时给予 ICI 可以通过产生一种"疫苗接种"效应引发临床上显著的抗肿瘤免疫反应，其机制为通过放疗诱导的细胞死亡暴露肿瘤抗原，这些肿瘤抗原可以被免疫系统识别并激活免疫反应，从而帮助免疫系统更有效地攻击和清除肿瘤细胞。然而，最近的研究表明，抗 PD-1 治疗与放疗之间的先后顺序可能会显著影响治疗效果。一项研究发现，在局部肿瘤放疗后使用抗 PD-1 抗体会导致肿瘤内的多功能 CD8+ T 细胞扩增，功能失调的 CD8+ T 细胞减少，以及可重编程的 CD8+ T 细胞的扩增。然而，在放疗前使用抗 PD-1 治疗，则会导致全身免疫功能下降，这主要是由于放射敏感性增加和 CD8+ T 细胞死亡[25]。

近年来，CD40 激动剂受到广泛关注，因其能使树突细胞（DC）激活辅助性 T 细胞反应，而辅助性 T 细胞反应对细胞毒性 CD8+ T 细胞的激活非常重要。CD40 是 TNF 受体家族的成员之一，在造血组织和非造血组织中均有表达。CD40L（CD154）主要由活化的 CD4+ T 淋巴细胞表达，它与 CD40 受体结合后，CD40 就会激活细胞。DC 上的 CD40 诱导共刺激分子配体（如 GITR、OX40 和 CD137）的表达增加，MHC

上调，IL-12 等促炎细胞因子产生，从而增强抗原呈递和适应性免疫激活。与前述放疗和 PD-1/PD-L1 抑制剂的联合使用类似，放疗也可与 CD40 激动剂联合使用。小鼠肿瘤模型实验表明，CD40 激活前给予 5~6 Gy 的单次低分割放疗剂量，产生协同作用的效果最佳[26]。该研究还表明，CD40 激动剂的疗效取决于 T 细胞和 BATF3-DC 的存在，而不依赖于 B 细胞和巨噬细胞。

在临床前试验中与放疗联用的另一类药物是 toll 样受体（toll-like receptor, TLR）激动剂。TLR 主要在免疫细胞上表达，在病原体感知和防御中发挥关键作用。这些受体依赖于病原体相关分子模式（pathogen-associated molecular pattern, PAMP）或内源性的损伤相关分子模式（damage-associated molecular pattern, DAMP），从而导致 APC 成熟和适应性免疫系统激活。最近的临床前研究表明，TLR 激动剂（特别是 TLR3、TLR9 和 TLR7/8）与放疗联合可能具有协同作用，增强抗肿瘤免疫应答[27]。这种效果归因于 TLR 激动剂在放疗后通过 DC 介导的 T 细胞激活增加。在正被评估的 TLR 激动剂中，TLR9 激动剂已在与 RT 联合使用的临床前模型中得到广泛研究。

5 HNSCC 放疗联合免疫治疗的临床评价

在临床环境中，放疗联合免疫治疗对于局部晚期、转移性或局部复发的肿瘤患者具有潜在的治疗获益价值。然而，在 HNSCC 患者中，获得有效的治疗反应所需的放疗最佳剂量、分割方式和联合治疗的时机在很大程度上仍是未知的。

PD-1 是一种免疫检查点受体，它与其配体 PD-L1（CD274）和 PD-L2（CD273）结合。在 HNSCC 中，无论是在 HPV 阳性还是 HPV 阴性肿瘤中，大多数效应 T 细胞都表达 PD-1 受体，在 HPV 阳性肿瘤中其表达水平相对更高[28]。研究发现在相当比例（46%~100%）的 HNSCC 中，PD-L1 蛋白表达较为普遍，而 PD-L2 蛋白表达较少，其主要局限在抗原呈递细胞上。尽管 PD-L2 在数量上较少，但它对 T 细胞产生的效应与 PD-L1 类似。CTLA-4 是首个临床靶向免疫检查点受体，主要在 T 细胞上表达，而在其他造血细胞类型上表达较少。迄今，抗 CTLA-4 抗体尚未被批准用于治疗 HNSCC，目前正在进行几项临床试验，评估将一种抗 CTLA-4 抗体（伊匹木单抗或替西木单抗）用于阻断 PD-1/PD-L1 途径（参见前面章节）[29]。

5.1 放疗联合免疫治疗用于转移性或复发性 HNSCC

在首例关于转移性 HNSCC 远隔效应的病例报告中，1 例肺转移患者在接受伊匹木单抗和纳武利尤单抗联合治疗后仍有进展，但在对原发性头颈部肿瘤病灶进行 3.7 Gy、每天 2 次、连续 2 天的姑息性放疗后，非照射区域的肺转移病灶出现部分缓解[30]。尽管该病例报告很有价值，但目前仍缺乏随机临床试验来阐明实现转移性 HNSCC 远隔效应的最佳治疗方案。临床前模型实验表明，低剂量分割放疗方案，如立体定向消融放疗（SABR）联合同步免疫治疗，可能是增强免疫激活的最佳策略。McBride 等（2021）首次报道了在转移性 HNSCC 中评估这种方法的 II 期随机试验。62 例转移性 HNSCC 患者（每例患者至少有 2 个转移灶）被随机分为 2 个治疗组：仅接受纳武利尤单抗治疗组（每 2 周 3 mg/kg，最长 96 周），与纳武利尤单抗联合单个转移灶放疗组（27 Gy，分 3 次，隔天 1 次）。主要终点是非照射区靶病灶的客观缓解率（objective response rate，ORR），次要终点包括总生存期（OS）和无进展生存期（PFS）。中位随访时间 20.2 个月后，仅使用纳武利尤单抗组的 ORR（34.5%）与纳武利尤单抗 +SABR 组（29%，P=0.86）之间没有差异。此外，两个治疗组的 PFS 和 OS 也没有统计学差异[31]。

有许多正在进行的试验研究免疫治疗和放疗在复发/转移性 HNSCC 中的联合应用，但大多数是小规模的探索性试验。我们将重点介绍一些研究，这些研究可能有助于我们优化放疗的剂量和分割方式，以及优化免疫治疗药物的选择。在一项正在进行的 II 期随机试验（NCT03386357）中，研究对象为一线铂类化疗失败的复发/转移性 HNSCC 患者，符合条件的对象被随机分为两组：帕博利珠单抗单药治疗组（每 3 周 200 mg）与帕博利珠单抗联合放疗组，放疗的靶病灶为 1~3 处转移病灶（36 Gy，分 12 次）。在联合治疗组中，帕博利珠单抗在第三次放疗剂量后开始，每 3 周 200 mg 持续使用直至 12 个月。主要终点是客观缓解率，次要终点包括缓解持续时间、无进展生存期、非放疗区靶病灶的大小变化、总生存期以及联合治疗的毒副反应。与 McBride 等（2021）的研究不同，这项 II 期试验在常规分割放疗方案下评估了帕博利珠单抗的疗效 [31]。

另一个值得注意的研究是一项 I/II 期单臂研究（NCT03283605）[32]，研究对象为有 2~10 个颅外寡转移灶的转移性 HNSCC 患者，该研究旨在评估度伐利尤单抗（每 4 周 1500 mg）与替西木单抗（每 4 周 75 mg，连续 4 个周期）和 SABR 联合治疗的安全性和疗效。所有受试者先接受 4 次剂量的度伐利尤单抗和替西木单抗后再单独接受度伐利尤单抗。SBRT 在度伐利尤单抗和替西木单抗的第 2 和第 3 周期之间进行。除了评估三联疗法的毒副反应外，该研究还将评估中位 OS 和远隔效应的发生率。

5.2 放疗联合免疫治疗用于局部晚期 HNSCC

在局部晚期 HNSCC（LA-HNSCC）患者中，高达 40% 的患者会发展为局部复发和（或）转移 [3-6]。目前仍有许多问题需要解决，包括如何将放疗与其他抗癌疗法（如化疗、手术）进行最佳结合，以及放疗最佳剂量、分割方式和时机选择等。尽管如此，利用放疗和免疫治疗之间的相互作用以改善患者治疗结果的实践一直在进行。

5.2.1 放疗联合免疫治疗用于不适用顺铂的患者

在一项 II 期单臂研究（NCT02609503）中，Weiss 等（2020）评估了帕博利珠单抗联合常规放疗治疗不适用顺铂的 LA-HNSCC 患者的疗效。患者接受 3 周期的帕博利珠单抗（每 3 周 200 mg），同期进行常规放疗（70 Gy，分 35 次），随后再接受 3 周期的帕博利珠单抗治疗。中位随访 21 个月，2 年的 PFS 和 OS 分别为 71% 和 75%。此外，观察到的毒副反应与仅进行放疗时预期的毒副反应相似，且 3 级和 4 级毒副作用较少 [33]。这项研究存在一些局限性，包括研究规模相对较小以及研究设计非随机化。这些因素可能会导致结果的偏差或无法得出明确的结论。首个随机 II 期试验（GORTEC 2015-01：NCT02707588）的结果已经公布，该试验评估了不适用顺铂的 LA-HNSCC 患者接受帕博利珠单抗与西妥昔单抗联合治疗的耐受性和安全性。患者被随机分配到两组：西妥昔单抗（400 mg/m² 负荷剂量，每周 250 mg/m²）联合同步放疗（69.96 Gy，分 33 次），或帕博利珠单抗（每 3 周 200 mg）联合同步放疗（69.96 Gy，分 33 次）。同步使用西妥昔单抗和放疗可观察到更高的 ≥ 3 级的毒副反应发生率，包括放射性皮炎和黏膜炎。而同步使用帕博利珠单抗和放疗组观察到较高的 ≥ 1 级的甲状腺功能异常发生率。中位随访 25.6 个月后，各治疗组的 2 年 PFS 和 OS 均没有差异。此外，15 个月时的局部控制率相似[34]。根据目前的情况，不适用顺铂的 LA-HNSCC 患者接受帕博利珠单抗联合常规放疗并不比西妥昔单抗联合常规放疗获得的生存率更高。然而，正如作者所建议的，可能需要更长的辅助免疫治疗时间，同时需要考虑使用的放疗剂量可能会对免疫激活产生负面影响。

5.2.2 同步放化疗与同期和辅助免疫治疗联合使用

Powell 等（2020）进行了一项 Ib 期临床试验（NCT02586207），评估了以顺铂为基础的同步放化疗联合帕博利珠单抗治疗 LA-HNSCC 患者的安全性和有效性。治疗方案包括在放化疗前 7 天静脉注射 200 mg 的帕博利珠单抗负荷剂量，放化疗期间在第 15 天和第 36 天各再注射 2 次，在完成后（巩固期）每 3 周注射 1 次，分别是第 57 天、第 78 天、第 99 天、第 120 天和第 141 天。放化疗从第 1 天开始，每周静脉注射顺铂 40 mg/m²，共 6 次计划剂量（最大总剂量为 240 mg/m²），同时进行头颈部调强放疗（IMRT），总剂量为 70 Gy，分 35 次进行，每日 1 次，每次 2 Gy。该治疗方案耐受性良好。根据 HPV 状态对患者进行分层，经过中位随访 28.4 个月后，HPV 阳性队列的 1 年和 2 年 OS 均为 97.1%。而对于 HPV 阴性患者，经过中位随访 17.5 个月后，1 年和 2 年的 OS 分别为 86.5% 和 53.1%[35]。

RTOG 3504 研究（NCT02764593）同样评估了纳武利尤单抗联合标准放化疗用于中高风险 LA-HNSCC 患者的安全性。患者被分配到 4 个治疗组：IMRT 联合纳武利尤单抗加每周给予顺铂组、IMRT 联合纳武利尤单抗加高剂量顺铂组、IMRT 联合西妥昔单抗组、IMRT 联合纳武利尤单抗组。关于安全性终点的初步报告显示，在同步化疗和 IMRT 的基础上加用纳武利尤单抗对新诊断的 LA-HNSCC 患者是安全的；但对接受高剂量顺铂或不适用顺铂的患者进行辅助性纳武利尤单抗治疗是不可行，由于药物的毒性反应和患者拒绝继续治疗，这两组中不到一半的患者完成了规定的 7 次纳武利尤单抗治疗[36]。

Ⅲ期临床试验 JAVELIN Head & Neck 100 研究（NCT02952586）评估了 LA-HNSCC 患者当前的标准治疗方案（高含剂量顺铂的放化疗）与抗 PD-L1 抗体阿维鲁单抗联合治疗的疗效。患者被随机分入 2 个治疗组（一个标准治疗组和一个试验组）：标准治疗组采用大剂量（100 mg/m^2）顺铂化疗同步放疗；试验组首次静脉注射负荷剂量的阿维鲁单抗（10 mg/kg），然后每 2 周给予 1 次阿维鲁单抗（10 mg/kg），并进行大剂量顺铂化疗同步放疗（70 Gy，分 35 次），最后再给予阿维鲁单抗（10 mg/kg）维持治疗 12 个月。主要终点是 PFS，次要终点包括 OS、ORR、DOR 和安全性。按计划进行中期分析后，该试验被认为无效，随后被终止，因为与标准治疗方案相比，试验组的 PFS 和 OS 并未改善[37-38]。尽管该方案效果不佳，但我们仍在等待Ⅲ期临床试验 KEYNOTE-412 研究（NCT03040999）的结果，该试验采用与 JAVELIN Head & Neck 100 研究相同的试验设计，但使用的是帕博利珠单抗治疗[39]。

5.2.3 同步放化疗与序贯免疫治疗相结合

根据已报道的随机临床试验，放疗或放化疗联合免疫治疗似乎对 LA-HNSCC 没有治疗效果。然而，在标准放化疗后进行序贯免疫治疗的方案已在非小细胞肺癌中显示生存获益，目前正在 LA-HNSCC 患者中进行评估[40]。与关于非小细胞肺癌的 PACIFIC 试验类似，许多正在进行的试验也在评估 HNSCC 在完成标准放化疗后进行序贯免疫治疗的获益情况。其中一项Ⅱ/Ⅲ期临床试验 ECOG ACRIN EA3161 研究（NCT03811015）评估了局部晚期 HPV 阳性中风险口咽癌患者进行标准放化疗后给予纳武利尤单抗维持治疗对 PFS 和 OS 的影响。放化疗结束后，患者被随机分配到治疗组（给予每 4 周 1 次的纳武利尤单抗，维持治疗 12 个月）或观察组[41]。PATHWay 研究（NCT02841748）是另一项正在进行中的随机Ⅱ期临床试验，在标准治疗后疾病复发风险≥40%~50% 的 HNSCC 患者中评估帕博利珠单抗辅助治疗对 PFS 的影响。患者被随机分配到帕博利珠单抗治疗组（每3周200 mg）和安慰剂组，持续治疗时间为12个月[42]。IMvoke010 研究是另一项Ⅲ期随机临床试验（NCT03452137），评估抗 PD-L1 抗体阿替利珠单抗单药治疗作为 HNSCC 标准治疗后的辅助治疗的效果。HPV 阳性和阴性的 HNSCC 患者接受标准治疗后被随机分配到安慰剂组或阿替利珠单抗治疗组（每3周1200 mg），治疗时间长达1年，主要研究终点包括无事件生存期和 OS[43]。

5.2.4 基于生物标志物的放疗与免疫检查点抑制剂联合使用

CHECKRAD-CD8 试验（NCT03426657）是一项在 LA-HNSCC 患者中开展的多中心Ⅱ期临床试验，该试验中放疗（70 Gy，分35次）和免疫检查抑制剂度伐利尤单抗与替西木单抗联合使用，然后再给予度伐利尤单抗维持治疗。在这项研究中，只有接受1周期诱导性顺铂、多西他赛、度伐利尤单抗和替西木单抗治疗后，肿瘤内 CD8+ T 细胞增加≥20% 或经组织病理学活检证实完全缓解（CR）的患者才继续接受上述联合治疗方案。其余患者则被排除出试验。在接受化疗免疫治疗诱导的79例患者中，41例患者（52%）获得了病理学 CR，31例（39%）患者出现肿瘤内 CD8+ T 细胞的增加，但未获得病理学 CR。在符合放疗联合免疫治疗条件的72例（91%）患者中，有60例完成了联合治疗。中位随访12.5个月，1年和2年的 PFS 分别为79%和73%，1年和2年的 OS 分别为89%和86%[44]。这种结合了生物标志物的研究设计，可以通过筛选出可能从这种治疗干预中获益的患者，从而实现放疗与免疫治疗的最佳联合。

6 其他有望与放疗联合使用的免疫药物

除了结合生物标志物来选择可能从放疗和免疫治疗的联合方案中获益的患者外，还有其他一些很有前景的方法可以进一步提高放疗联合免疫治疗的疗效。加强它们协同作用的一个有效途径是添加小分子表观遗传调节剂，如组蛋白去乙酰化酶（histone deacetylase, HDAC）抑制剂（图 6-2），特别是在 R/M HNSCC 患者中。在临床前模型实验中，HDAC 抑制剂可上调 MHC Ⅰ、MHC Ⅱ 和 CD40 的表达。一项 Ⅱ 期临床试验显示，HDAC 抑制剂 vorinostat 和帕博利珠单抗联合治疗 R/M HNSCC 的缓解率为 32%，而据报道帕博利珠单抗单药的缓解率仅为 18%[45]。由于放疗和 HDAC 抑制剂能增强肿瘤的免疫应答和抗原呈递，因此将这两种疗法与免疫治疗相结合可能是克服肿瘤对免疫治疗耐药机制的有效方法。目前，美国 FDA 批准的免疫治疗药物主要以 T 细胞为靶点；然而，NK 细胞是先天性免疫系统的关键效应器，能够杀死缺乏 MHC Ⅰ 的恶性肿瘤细胞，而无须预先致敏，因此可以快速激发抗肿瘤活性。研究发现，包括 HNSCC 在内的多种恶性肿瘤中，NK 细胞在肿瘤组织间质中的浸润与患者的生存相关[46]。因此，增强 NK 细胞在 HNSCC TME 中的浸润和细胞毒性可能是一种有前景的治疗方法，可与放疗联合使用。

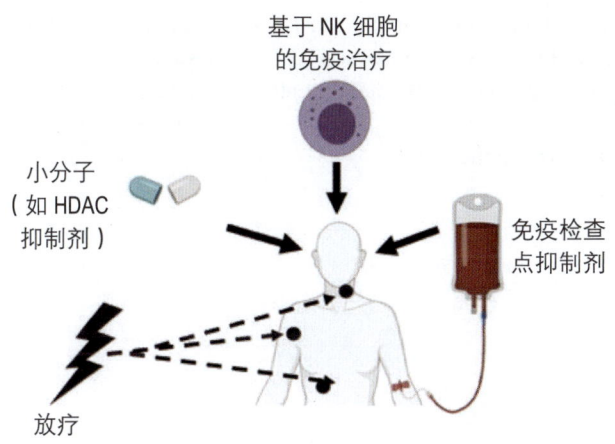

图 6-2 转移性或复发性头颈部鳞状细胞癌强化免疫治疗的建议策略。对所有病灶进行放疗可以减轻肿瘤负荷并增强免疫治疗药物的治疗效果。小分子药物，如表观遗传调节剂（HDAC 抑制剂），具有免疫刺激作用，包括上调 MHC Ⅰ 和 MHC Ⅱ。因此，它们可以与放疗联合使用，以克服免疫治疗药物的原发性和继发性耐药。靶向 NK 细胞等先天性免疫系统是一种有前景的免疫治疗方法，可作为单药治疗或与放疗及其他肿瘤治疗方式联合使用，以获得最佳的治疗效果[45-47]。

7 结论

尽管免疫治疗药物取得了成功，但仍存在许多挑战，包括缓解率低和产生耐药性[111]。放疗可以作为克服这些挑战的一种手段，以充分发挥免疫治疗的临床疗效。然而，关于放疗剂量、分割方式、范围和最佳联合方式等问题仍未得到解答。希望正在进行的试验（表6-1）能在不久的将来部分解决其中的一些问题。我们的研究重点应从探索如何实现罕见的远隔效应，转变为将放疗作为一种细胞减灭疗法，即通过减少肿瘤细胞数量来增强免疫治疗的效果。鉴于SABR-COMET试验的结果，以及免疫治疗可能对低肿瘤负荷患者更有效的观点[21, 47]，放疗与免疫治疗的联合对于寡转移灶患者的治疗可能是最有前景的。

原文符合伦理标准相关声明

Disclosure of Potential Conflicts of Interest   Quaovi H. Sodji and Dhanya K. Nambiar declare that they have no conflict of interest.

Quaovi H. Sodji is supported by the Kaplan Fellowship from the Department of Radiation Oncology at Stanford University. Quynh Thu Le and Dhanya K. Nambiar are supported by 5 R01 DE029672-02. Quynh Thu Le has served as a consultant for Nanobiotix, Merck Sharp Dome and on an advisory board for Roche/Genentech, Coherus, and Grail in the last 3 years.

Informed Consent   Not applicable.

表 6-1 研究头颈部鳞状细胞癌放疗与免疫检查点抑制剂联合使用的部分试验

临床试验	临床分期	疾病状态	治疗方案	放疗分割方案	组合顺序	试验状态/结果	参考文献
NCT02684253	II期随机	转移性	纳武利尤单抗，每2周，共96周	SABR（27 Gy，隔天，3次）	同步治疗	无差异	McBride et al.[31]
NCT03386357	II期随机	复发和（或）转移性	帕博利珠单抗，每3周	常规放疗（36 Gy，12次）	同步治疗	进行中	Clinical-trials.gov
NCT03283605	I/II期，单臂	转移性	度伐利尤单抗（每4周，直到疾病进展）和替西木单抗（每4周，4个周期）	SABR	免疫治疗→放疗→免疫治疗	进行中	Bahig et al.[32]
NCT02609503	II期，单臂	LA-HNSCC	帕博利珠单抗，每3周，共6个周期	常规放疗（70 Gy，35次）	同步治疗+辅助治疗	2年 OS：75%，2年 PFS：71%	Weiss et al.[33]
NCT02707588 GORTE 2015-01 (PembroRad)	II期随机	LA-HNSCC	帕博利珠单抗，每3周，共3个周期	常规放疗（69.96 Gy，33次）	同步治疗	两组2年OS和PFS无显著差异	Bourhis et al.[34]
NCT02586207	Ib期，单臂	LA-HNSCC	帕博利珠单抗，每3周，共8个周期	常规放疗（70 Gy，35次）	初始免疫治疗→同步免疫治疗+放化疗→辅助免疫治疗	2年 OS： • HPV(+)：97.1% • HPV(−)：53.1%	Powell et al.[35]
NCT02764593 (RTOG 3504)	I期，非随机	LA-HNSCC	纳武利尤单抗	常规放疗（70 Gy，35次）	同步治疗+辅助治疗	同时纳武利尤单抗化疗与放疗安全	Gillison et al.[36]

（续表）

临床试验	临床分期	疾病状态	治疗方案	放疗分割方案	组合顺序	试验状态/结果	参考文献
NCT02952586（JAVELIN Head & Neck 100）	Ⅲ期随机	LA-HNSCC	阿维鲁单抗，每2周，共12个月	常规放疗（70 Gy，35次）	初始免疫治疗→同步免疫治疗+放化疗→辅助免疫治疗	阴性：实验组与安慰剂组 OS 和 PFS 无差异	Lee et al. [38]
NCT03040999（KEYNOTE-412）	Ⅲ期随机	LA-HNSCC	帕博利珠单抗，每3周，共17个周期	常规放疗（70 Gy，35次）	初始免疫治疗→同步免疫治疗+放化疗→辅助免疫治疗	进行中	Machiels et al. [39]
NCT03811015（ECOG ACRIN EA3161）	Ⅱ/Ⅲ期随机	局部晚期 HPV（+）OPSCC	纳武利尤单抗，每4周，共12个月	常规放疗（70 Gy，35次）	辅助治疗	进行中	Saba et al. [41]
NCT02841748（PATHWay Study）	Ⅱ期随机	HNSCC（复发风险≥40%～50%）	帕博利珠单抗，每3周，共1年	常规放疗（根治性放疗）	辅助治疗	进行中	Bauml et al. [42]
NCT03452137（IMvoke010）	Ⅲ期随机	LA-HNSCC	阿替利珠单抗，每3周，共1年	常规放疗（根治性放疗）	辅助治疗	进行中	Haddad et al. [43]
NCT03426657	Ⅱ期单臂	LA-HNSCC	度伐利尤单抗和替西木单抗，每4周，共4个周期；随后度伐利尤单抗维持治疗，共8个周期	常规放疗（根治性放疗）	诱导双免疫治疗→同时放疗+双免疫治疗→维持免疫治疗	2年 PFS：73%，2年 OS：86%	Hecht et al. [44]

HPV：人乳头瘤病毒；OPSCC：口咽鳞状细胞癌；OS：总生存期；PFS：无进展生存期；SABR：立体定向消融放射治疗

参考文献

1. Siegel RL, Miller KD, Jemal A (2020) Cancer statistics, 2020. CA Cancer J Clin 70:7-30. https://doi.org/10.3322/caac.21590
2. Bray F, Ferlay J, Soerjomataram I et al (2018) Global cancer statistics 2018: GLOBOCAN estimates of incidence and mortality worldwide for 36 cancers in 185 countries. CA Cancer J Clin 68:394-424. https://doi.org/10.3322/caac.21492
3. Marur S, Forastiere AA (2016) Head and neck squamous cell carcinoma: update on epidemiology, diagnosis, and treatment. Mayo Clin Proc 91:386-396. https://doi.org/10.1016/j.mayocp.2015.12.017
4. Cognetti DM, Weber RS, Lai SY (2008) Head and neck cancer: an evolving treatment paradigm. Cancer 113:1911-1932. https://doi.org/10.1002/cncr.23654
5. Vermorken JB, Specenier P (2010) Optimal treatment for recurrent/metastatic head and neck cancer. Ann Oncol 21:vii252-vii261. https://doi.org/10.1093/annonc/mdq453
6. Marur S, Forastiere AA (2008) Head and neck cancer: changing epidemiology, diagnosis, and treatment. Mayo Clin Proc 83:489-501. https://doi.org/10.4065/83.4.489
7. Kaufman HL, Atkins MB, Subedi P et al (2019) The promise of Immuno-oncology: implications for defining the value of cancer treatment. J Immunother Cancer. https://doi.org/10.1186/s40425-019-0594-0
8. Bhat AA, Yousuf P, Wani NA et al (2021) Tumor microenvironment: an evil nexus promoting aggressive head and neck squamous cell carcinoma and avenue for targeted therapy. Signal Transduct Target Ther. https://doi.org/10.1038/s41392-021-00503-9
9. Mandal R, Şenbabaoğlu Y, Desrichard A et al (2016) The head and neck cancer immune landscape and its immunotherapeutic implications. JCI Insight. https://doi.org/10.1172/jci.insight.89829
10. de Ruiter EJ, Ooft ML, Devriese LA et al (2017) The prognostic role of tumor infiltrating T-lymphocytes in squamous cell carcinoma of the head and neck: a systematic review and meta-analysis. Oncoimmunology. https://doi.org/10.1080/2162402X.2017.1356148
11. Fares CM, Van Allen EM, Drake CG et al (2019) Mechanisms of resistance to immune checkpoint blockade: why does checkpoint inhibitor immunotherapy not work for all patients? Am Soc Clin Oncol Educ Book 39:147-164. https://doi.org/10.1200/EDBK_240837
12. Chan TA, Yarchoan M, Jaffee E et al (2019) Development of tumor mutation burden as an immunotherapy biomarker: utility for the oncology clinic. Ann Oncol 30:44-56. https://doi.org/10.1093/annonc/mdy495
13. McCulloch HD (1908) On the analogy between spontaneous recoveries from cancer and the specific immunity induced by X ray irradiations of the lymphatic glands involved. Br Med J 2:1146-1148. https://doi.org/10.1136/bmj.2.2494.1146
14. Bentzen SM, Harari PM, Bernier J (2007) Exploitable mechanisms for combining drugs with radiation: concepts, achievements and future directions. Nat Clin Pract Oncol 4:172-180. https://doi.org/10.1038/ncponc0744
15. Golden EB, Apetoh L (2015) Radiotherapy and immunogenic cell death. Semin Radiat Oncol 25:11-17. https://doi.org/10.1016/j.semradonc.2014.07.005
16. Reits EA, Hodge JW, Herberts CA et al (2006) Radiation modulates the peptide repertoire, enhances MHC class I expression, and induces successful antitumor immunotherapy. J Exp Med

203:1259-1271. https://doi.org/10.1084/jem.20052494
17. Gasser S, Orsulic S, Brown EJ et al (2005) The DNA damage pathway regulates innate immune system ligands of the NKG2D receptor. Nature 436:1186-1190. https://doi.org/10.1038/nature03884
18. Deng L, Liang H, Burnette B et al (2014) Irradiation and anti-PD-L1 treatment synergistically promote antitumor immunity in mice. J Clin Invest 124:687-695. https://doi.org/10.1172/JCI67313
19. Schaue D, Kachikwu EL, McBride WH (2012) Cytokines in radiobiological responses: a review. Radiat Res 178:505-523. https://doi.org/10.1667/RR3031.1
20. Seiwert TY, Kiess AP (2021) Time to debunk an urban myth? The "abscopal effect" with radiation and anti-PD-1. J Clin Oncol 39:1-3. https://doi.org/10.1200/JCO.20.02046
21. Palma DA, Olson R, Harrow S et al (2019) Stereotactic ablative radiotherapy versus standard of care palliative treatment in patients with oligometastatic cancers (SABR-COMET): a randomised, phase 2, open-label trial. Lancet 393:2051-2058. https://doi.org/10.1016/S0140-6736(18)32487-5
22. Sridharan V, Margalit DN, Lynch SA et al (2016) Definitive chemoradiation alters the immunologic landscape and immune checkpoints in head and neck cancer. Br J Cancer 115:252-260. https://doi.org/10.1038/bjc.2016.166
23. Verbrugge I, Hagekyriakou J, Sharp LL et al (2012) Radiotherapy increases the permissiveness of established mammary tumors to rejection by immunomodulatory antibodies. Cancer Res 72:3163-3174. https://doi.org/10.1158/0008-5472. CAN-12-0210
24. Dovedi SJ, Adlard AL, Lipowska-Bhalla G et al (2014) Acquired resistance to fractionated radiotherapy can be overcome by concurrent PD-L1 blockade. Cancer Res 74:5458-5468. https://doi.org/10.1158/0008-5472. CAN-14-1258
25. Wei J, Montalvo-Ortiz W, Yu L et al (2021) Sequence of αPD-1 relative to local tumor irradiation determines the induction of abscopal antitumor immune responses. Sci Immunol. https://doi.org/10.1126/sciimmunol.abg0117
26. Yasmin-Karim S, Bruck PT, Moreau M et al (2018) Radiation and local anti-CD40 generate an effective in situ vaccine in preclinical models of pancreatic cancer. Front Immunol. https://doi.org/10.3389/fimmu.2018.02030
27. Marabelle A, Filatenkov A, Sagiv-Barfi I et al (2015) Radiotherapy and toll-like receptor agonists. Semin Radiat Oncol 25:34-39. https://doi.org/10.1016/j.semradonc.2014.07.006
28. Badoual C, Hans S, Merillon N et al (2013) PD-1-expressing tumor-infiltrating T cells are a favorable prognostic biomarker in HPV-associated head and neck cancer. Cancer Res 73:128-138. https://doi.org/10.1158/0008-5472. CAN-12-2606
29. Ferris RL, Haddad R, Even C et al (2020) Durvalumab with or without tremelimumab in patients with recurrent or metastatic head and neck squamous cell carcinoma: EAGLE, a randomized, open-label phase III study. Ann Oncol 31:942-950. https://doi.org/10.1016/j.annonc.2020.04.001
30. Shinde A, Novak J, Freeman ML et al (2019) Induction of the abscopal effect with immunotherapy and palliative radiation in metastatic head and neck squamous cell carcinoma: a case report and review of the literature. Cureus. https://doi.org/10.7759/cureus.4201
31. McBride S, Sherman E, Tsai CJ et al (2021) Randomized phase II trial of nivolumab with stereotactic body radiotherapy versus nivolumab alone in metastatic head and neck squamous cell carcinoma. J Clin Oncol 39:30-37. https://doi.org/10.1200/JCO.20.00290
32. Bahig H, Aubin F, Stagg J et al (2019) Phase I/II trial of durvalumab plus tremelimumab and

stereotactic body radiotherapy for metastatic head and neck carcinoma. BMC Cancer. https://doi.org/10.1186/s12885-019-5266-4
33. Weiss J, Sheth S, Deal AM et al (2020) Concurrent definitive immunoradiotherapy for patients with stage III-IV head and neck cancer and cisplatin contraindication. Clin Cancer Res 26:4260-4267. https://doi.org/10.1158/1078-0432. CCR-20-0230
34. Bourhis J, Sire C, Tao Y et al (2020) LBA38 pembrolizumab versus cetuximab, concomitant with radiotherapy (RT) in locally advanced head and neck squamous cell carcinoma (LA-HNSCC): results of the GORTEC 2015-01 "PembroRad" randomized trial. Ann Oncol. https://doi.org/10.1016/j.annonc.2020.08.2268
35. Powell SF, Gold KA, Gitau MM et al (2020) Safety and efficacy of pembrolizumab with chemoradiotherapy in locally advanced head and neck squamous cell carcinoma: a phase IB study. J Clin Oncol 38:2427-2437. https://doi.org/10.1200/JCO.19.03156
36. Gillison ML, Ferris RL, Harris J et al (2019) Safety and disease control achieved with the addition of nivolumab (Nivo) to chemoradiotherapy (CRT) for intermediate (IR) and high-risk (HR) local-regionally advanced head and neck squamous cell carcinoma (HNSCC): RTOG Foundation 3504. J Clin Oncol. https://doi.org/10.1200/JCO.2019.37.15_suppl.6073
37. Cohen EE, Ferris RL, Psyrri A et al (2020) 910O Primary results of the phase III JAVELIN head & neck 100 trial: Avelumab plus chemoradiotherapy (CRT) followed by avelumab maintenance vs CRT in patients with locally advanced squamous cell carcinoma of the head and neck (LA SCCHN). Ann Oncol. https://doi.org/10.1016/j.annonc.2020.08.1025
38. Lee NY, Ferris RL, Psyrri A et al (2021) Avelumab plus standard-of-care chemoradiotherapy versus chemoradiotherapy alone in patients with locally advanced squamous cell carcinoma of the head and neck: a randomised, double-blind, placebo-controlled, multicentre, phase 3 trial. Lancet Oncol 22:450-462. https://doi.org/10.1016/S1470-2045(20)30737-3
39. Machiels J-P, Tao Y, Burtness B et al (2020) Pembrolizumab given concomitantly with chemoradiation and as maintenance therapy for locally advanced head and neck squamous cell carcinoma: KEYNOTE-412. Future Oncol 16:1235-1243. https://doi.org/10.2217/fon-2020-0184
40. Antonia SJ, Villegas A, Daniel D et al (2017) Durvalumab after chemoradiotherapy in stage III non-small-cell lung cancer. N Engl J Med 377:1919-1929. https://doi.org/10.1056/NEJMoa1709937
41. Saba NF, Li S, Hussain ZA et al (2018) Locally advanced high-risk HPV related oropharyngeal squamous cell carcinoma (OPSCC); have we forgotten it is a different disease? Cancers Head Neck. https://doi.org/10.1186/s41199-018-0035-7
42. Bauml J, Karrison T, Vokes EE et al (2017) A randomized, double-blind phase II study of pembrolizumab versus placebo in patients with head and neck cancers at high risk for recurrence or low-volume residual disease: the PATHWay study. J Clin Oncol. https://doi.org/10.1200/JCO.2017.35.15_suppl.TPS6095
43. Haddad R, Wong DJ, Guo Y et al (2018) 1117TiP-IMvoke010: randomized phase III study of atezolizumab (atezo) as adjuvant monotherapy after definitive therapy of squamous cell carcinoma of the head and neck (SCCHN). Ann Oncol. https://doi.org/10.1093/annonc/mdy287
44. Hecht M, Eckstein M, Rutzner S et al (2021) Primary results of the phase II CheckRad-CD8 trial: first-line treatment of locally advanced head and neck squamous cell carcinoma (HNSCC) with double checkpoint blockade and radiotherapy dependent on intratumoral CD8+ T-cell infiltration. J Clin Oncol. https://doi.org/10.1200/JCO.2021.39.15_suppl.6007

45. Rodriguez CP, Wu QV, Voutsinas J et al (2020) A phase II trial of pembrolizumab and vorinostat in recurrent metastatic head and neck squamous cell carcinomas and salivary gland cancer. Clin Cancer Res 26:837-845. https://doi.org/10.1158/1078-0432. CCR-19-2214
46. Russick J, Torset C, Hemery E et al (2020) NK cells in the tumor microenvironment: prognostic and theranostic impact. Recent advances and trends. Semin Immunol. https://doi.org/10.1016/j.smim.2020.101407
47. Arina A, Gutiontov SI, Weichselbaum RR (2020) Radiotherapy and immunotherapy for cancer: from "systemic" to "multisite". Clin Cancer Res 26:2777-2782. https://doi.org/10.1158/1078-0432. CCR-19-2034

第7章 免疫治疗在头颈部肿瘤围术期管理中的临床应用

Clinical Application of Immunotherapy in the Perioperative Management of Head and Neck Cancer

（Frederick M. Howard, Nishant Agrawal, Ari J. Rosenberg 著）
（韩光，袁程，徐璐，易廷庄 译）

> **摘要**
>
> 免疫治疗改变了复发/转移头颈部鳞状细胞癌的治疗现状，现已成为此类患者一线系统治疗的重要手段。临床研究已开始评估围术期的免疫治疗，包括免疫检查点抑制剂（ICI）单药或与化疗联合使用，或将

原作者信息

F. M. Howard
Section of Hematology/Oncology, Department of Medicine, The University of Chicago Medicine and Biological Sciences, Chicago, IL, USA
e-mail: Frederick.howard2@uchospitals.edu

N. Agrawal
Otolaryngology-Head and Neck Surgery, The University of Chicago Medicine, Chicago, IL, USA

Head and Neck Surgical Oncology, The University of Chicago Medicine, Chicago, IL, USA
Surgery, Radiation Oncology, Comprehensive Cancer Center, The University of Chicago Pritzker School of Medicine, Chicago, IL, USA
e-mail: na@uchicago.edu

A. J. Rosenberg (✉)
Section of Hematology/Oncology, Department of Medicine, The University of Chicago Medicine, Chicago, IL, USA
e-mail: arirosenberg@medicine.bsd.uchicago.edu

ICI 与其他免疫调节剂联合使用。不断有研究表明，免疫治疗产生的病理反应可改善患者的长期预后，且不会延迟手术。但目前有多种不同的方法用于量化试验中的治疗反应，因此需要统一方法。据报道，新辅助化疗免疫治疗的疗效尤为显著，两项小型研究显示，约 2/3 的 HPV 阳性患者获得了完全缓解。评估围术期 ICI 单药治疗的几项研究表明，PD-L1 的表达会增强免疫治疗的获益。虽然早期数据很可观，但并非所有患者都对免疫治疗有反应。目前，一些研究正在进行中，旨在发现或确定预测生物标志物、新的免疫检查点靶点，或能提高疗效的免疫调节剂联合疗法。围术期研究为科学发现提供了理想渠道，因为其可以利用基线组织和术后切除的肿瘤进行相关研究。

关键词

辅助性免疫检查点阻断·免疫检查点抑制剂·头颈部恶性肿瘤·头颈部鳞状细胞癌·免疫治疗·新辅助治疗·围术期

1 引言

头颈部恶性肿瘤常为局部晚期肿瘤，经典治疗方法包括手术和（或）放化疗，许多患者需要三联疗法以达到治愈目的。尽管进行了积极的多模式治疗，但只有一半以上的 HPV 阴性患者和 80%~90% 的 HPV 阳性患者能在确诊后存活 5 年[1]。有少量文献支持首选外科手术或以放疗为基础的治疗方案，其中一些研究结果倾向于支持对于口腔癌患者首选外科手术[2]，而另一些研究则显示无论采用哪种方法，长期疗效均相当[3]。因此，治疗方案的选择在很大程度上取决于手术切除的可行性、患者的身体状况以及通过手术或放射治疗所能够达到的功能性结果。

新辅助治疗或诱导治疗已被探索用于改善头颈部鳞状细胞癌患者的功能结局，主要通过减少手术范围[4]或避免全喉切除术[5]。此外，诱导化疗的疗效也可作为后续治疗减量的依据[6]。然而，新辅助治疗对患者长期预后的具体影响尚不明确。同样，多个关于非手术治疗前诱导化疗的随机对照试验表明，诱导化疗可降低远处转移的风险，但其在最佳同步放化疗前的生存获益仍存在争议[7]。

随着新的有效化疗药物的研发[8]，诱导治疗方案在不断发展，免疫治疗在转移性肿瘤中的应用范围也在不断扩展，促使人们开始探索在治愈性治疗方案中应用免疫疗法。新辅助治疗在对免疫治疗有反应的其他肿瘤中也已取得成功[9-11]。在乳腺癌和肺癌的新辅助化疗中，根据PD-L1状态并不能完全确定哪些患者可从免疫治疗中获益，说明转移性肿瘤的生物标志物并不一定适用于早期疾病。随着更大规模的HNSCC围术期免疫治疗试验的完成，对来自转移性环境的生物标志物进行严格评估将变得非常重要。

2 疗效评估

新辅助治疗模式能够在早期肿瘤中对新治疗药物进行快速评估。由于新辅助治疗可以在治疗过程中观察患者的治疗反应，提供对治疗方案的早期反馈，并且能够在手术时采集相关的生物标志物，因此可以迅速评估药物的有效性和安全性。在新辅助治疗中应用免疫治疗的临床试验通常会采用病理学或影像学评估作为主要或次要的评价指标，这些评价指标已在诱导化疗试验中被证实具有预后价值。其他用于评估免疫治疗疗效的新指标还在开发中。

2.1 病理反应疗效评估

越来越多的证据表明，病理反应可以作为长期生存的一个重要替代性指标。在美国退伍军人事务部喉部研究（Veterans Affairs Larynx Study）项目中，101例患者在顺铂和5-FU诱导化疗后接受了活检，其中有病理残留的患者4年无病生存率（disease-free survival, DFS）<30%，而无肿瘤残留患者的无病生存率近80%[12]。在Licitra等（2003）发表的研究结果中，98例可手术切除的口腔鳞状细胞癌患者随机接受顺铂+5-FU诱导化疗，病理学完全缓解（pathologic complete response, pCR）或显微镜下有残留病灶（散在的少量病灶）的患者5年DFS明显

高于有残留病灶的患者（85%对比49%，$P=0.001$）[4]。因此，HNSCC新辅助化疗的病理反应是一个早已明确的替代终点，用于评估治疗效果和预测患者的长期生存情况。然而，目前仅有一些初步数据表明免疫治疗反应与长期预后之间存在类似关系。

尽管如此，人们还是开发出了各种评价指标来更好地量化治疗反应。主要病理学缓解（major pathologic response, MPR）是指新辅助治疗后瘤床内残存活肿瘤细胞的百分比≤10%，无论淋巴结内有无活肿瘤细胞残存，其长期以来一直被认为是NSCLC新辅助化疗后的替代性预后指标[13]。对免疫治疗有反应的患者具有一些特征，例如免疫浸润区退化，伤口愈合和细胞死亡方面也有一些特征，提示对免疫治疗进行评估需要有更多考虑到这些特征的新评价标准。因此，免疫相关病理反应标准（immune-related pathologic response criteria, irPRC）应运而生，该标准根据肿瘤消退和坏死区域的比例对肿瘤床进行量化，有更高的观察者间一致性[14]。

尽管在HNSCC中需要严格的统一性标准来描述患者对免疫治疗的反应，并且这些标准需要有经过验证的预后价值，但最近的几项试验利用irPRC的残留肿瘤床概念对HNSCC的病理学肿瘤缓解（pathologic tumor response, pTR）进行分类[15-16]。pTR是残留肿瘤的倒数，其定义为病理学缓解（肿瘤坏死、角质碎片和巨细胞/组织细胞反应）区域在病理学缓解区域和存活肿瘤之和中所占的比例。根据缓解区域所占的百分比进一步分类为pTR-0（＜10%，反应差）、pTR-1（10%～49%）和pTR-2（≥50%，反应良好）。据报道，术前使用帕博利珠单抗的一项Ⅲ期临床试验（NCT03765918）正在评估pTR的预后价值[16]，其他试验也采用了等效的评分系统，将pTR≥90%定义为主要病理学缓解（MPR），pTR≥20%定义为部分病理学缓解（partial pathologic response, PPR），pTR＜20%定义为无病理学缓解（no pathologic response, NPR）（图7-1）。病理学缓解对于化疗的预后意义已经确定，对于免疫治疗而言，虽然初步数据提示免疫治疗的病理学缓解是复发的替代终点，但还需要对缓解进行统一量化。

图 7-1 新辅助免疫治疗研究的病理学缓解评估标准

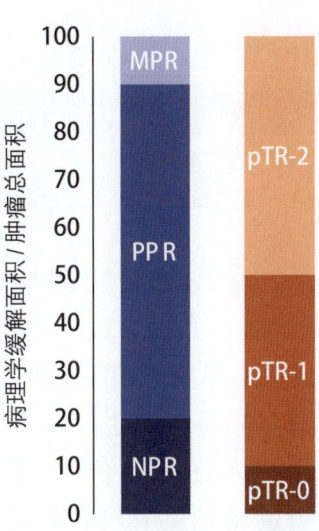

2.2 影像学疗效评估

有几项新辅助免疫治疗试验使用了细胞毒性化疗评估中用的影像学反应作为评估终点。因为 HNSCC 的形状不规则，WHO 标准和 RECIST 标准都存在局限性，并且与病理反应的相关性较差[17]。为了解决这一问题，有研究者提出通过体积反应进行评估，但目前还缺乏在接受诱导化疗患者中的长期试验结果来证实其有效性[18]。

免疫治疗进一步增加了通过影像学反应进行评估的挑战性，因为肿瘤大小会受到炎症浸润和纤维化的干扰，从而影响评估结果[14]。修订后的 WHO 标准和 RECIST 标准 [即免疫相关反应标准（irRC）和免疫相关 RECIST 标准（irRECIST）] 已在不同组织学类型中被用于评估免疫治疗的临床获益，这两个标准皆建议确认肿瘤生长情况或是否出现新的靶病灶，对于病情处于进展边缘的患者更格外需要确认[19]。假性进展在 HNC 中相对罕见，然而在 CHECKMATE-141 研究中，有 1.3% 的患者开始时被认为病情进展，但后来出现了缓解[20]。因此，使用影像学反应标准来评估新辅助免疫治疗的益处尚不明确，没有任何反应标准能充分应对因肿瘤床炎症消退而在影像学上出现残留病灶的患者。为了尽量避免延误根治性治疗，术前免疫治疗时间一般都很短暂，因此进行连续成像检查可能不切实际。此外，对于化疗联合免疫治疗而言，影像学反应可能与病理学完全缓解的相关性较差[21]。因此影像学反应在新辅助治疗试验中的作用仍有待明确。

3　免疫检查点抑制剂单药治疗

一些不同的围术期免疫治疗方案已经或正在被评估用于治疗 HNSCC（图 7-2）。有两项 Ⅱ 期临床试验获得了在新辅助和辅助治疗中使用帕博利珠单抗治疗 HPV 阴性肿瘤的初步数据（表 7-1）。Uppaluri 及其同事报道了一项多中心 Ⅱ 期临床试验（NCT02296684）的结果，该试验评估了 36 例 Ⅲ~Ⅳb 期（根据 AJCC 第 7 版）HPV 阴性 HNSCC 患者的新辅助和辅助治疗应用帕博利珠单抗的结果[16]。帕博利珠单抗在原发性肿瘤切除和同侧/对侧颈部淋巴结清扫术前 13~22 天给药，其中具有淋巴结外浸润或切缘阳性的患者接受术后放化疗，随后接受 6 个周期的帕博利珠单抗治疗，而其他患者则根据医生的建议接受观察、RT 或放化疗。其中有 18 例（50%）具有高风险特征（淋巴结外浸润或切缘阳性）的患者接受了辅助放化疗，并在术后 3 个月开始接受额外 6 个周期的帕博利珠单抗治疗，有 6 例患者由于放化疗毒性反应未恢复而未接受帕博利珠单抗治疗；低风险患者则接受辅助放化疗、单纯 RT 或随访观察。在高风险患者中，主要终点 1 年复发率为 16.7%（95%CI：3.6%~41.4%），与既往接受类似治疗的患者（复发率约为 35%）相比，显示有治疗获益[22]；低风险患者 1 年内无复发。然而，由于该临床试验预计将招募更多具有高风险特征的患者，因此，对试验方案进行了修订后，增加了 pTR-2 作为共同主要终点，修订后显示 22% 的患者出现了 pTR-2，pTR-1 及 pTR-2 患者 1 年内无复发，而 pTR-0（无应答）患者的复发率为 16%。鉴于样本量较小且存在混杂因素的可能性，需谨慎理解 pTR 的预后价值。在该试验中，帕博利珠单抗新辅助治疗未出现 3~4 级免疫相关不良事件，手术或辅助治疗也未出现意外延迟。多项相关性分析显示，通过多重免疫荧光评估的肿瘤细胞 PD-L1 阳性率（$r=0.42$，95%CI：0.08~0.67）和 CD8+ 细胞数（$r=0.72$，95%CI：0.44~0.88）与 pTR 呈正相关，而肿瘤突变负荷和预测的新抗原负荷则不相关。在 pTR 患者中，免疫相关基因和炎症因子（包括 IFNG、

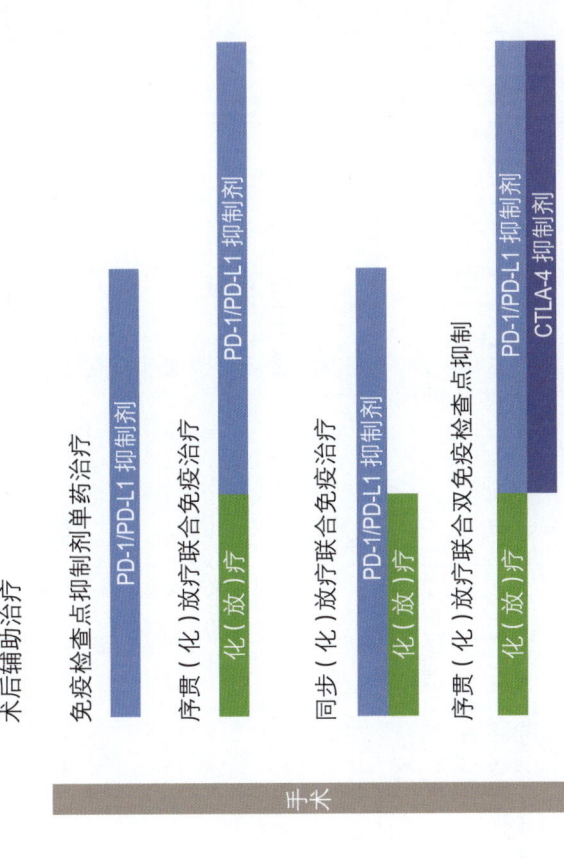

图 7-2 头颈部鳞状细胞癌围术期免疫检查点抑制策略示例

表 7-1 关于围术期免疫检查点阻断免疫治疗已完成的试验及初步数据

临床试验	患者入组标准	治疗方案	样本量	缓解率	复发率
NCT02296684 II 期	III/IV 期，HPV 阴性	帕博利珠单抗 ×1→手术→(C)RT/观察→若高风险则帕博利珠单抗 ×6	36[a]	pTR-2: 22%；pTR-1: 22%；pTR-0: 56%	1 年 DFS: 91%； 高风险：1 年 DFS: 82%； 低风险：1 年 DFS: 91%
NCT02641093 II 期	T3~T4 或 2 个以上阳性淋巴结，HPV 阴性	帕博利珠单抗 ×1→手术→帕博利珠单抗 ×6+(C)RT（高风险时每周顺铂）	76	MPR: 4%；PPR: 39%；NPR: 57%	高风险：1 年 DFS: 68%； 中风险：1 年 DFS: 97%
NCT03021993 II 期	II~IVA 期，口腔癌	纳武利尤单抗 ×3~4→手术	9[a]	PR[b]: 44%；SD: 11%；PD: 44%	3 例复发
NCT02488759 (CheckMate 358) I/II 期	T1+ 和 N1+	纳武利尤单抗 ×2→手术	12 HPV+；17 HPV-	PR (RECIST): HPV+: 50%；HPV-: 46%	N/A
NCT03355560 II 期	放疗后复发	手术→纳武利尤单抗 ×6	39	N/A	2 年 DFS: 60%
NCT03341936 II 期	可切除复发性疾病，病程间隔 >8 周	纳武利尤单抗 +lirilumab ×1→手术→纳武利尤单抗 +lirilumab ×6	5 HPV+；23 HPV-	pTR-2: 14%；pTR-1: 29%；pTR-0: 57%	1 年 DFS: 55.2%
NCT03565783 II 期	III/IV 期，皮肤头颈部鳞癌	西米普利单抗 ×2→手术	20	影像学： PR (RECIST): 30%； SD (RECIST): 60%； 病理学： pCR: 55%；MPR: 15%	手术+放化疗后 1 例疾病进展

（续表）

临床试验	患者入组标准	治疗方案	样本量	缓解率	复发率
NCT03057613 Ⅱ期	皮肤头颈部 SCC，T4、淋巴结阳性或高风险	手术→IMRT+帕博利珠单抗×16	18	N/A	N/A
NCT02919683 Ⅱ期随机	口腔癌 T2~T4b 或 N+	第1组：纳武利尤单抗×2→手术	14	MPR：8%；pTR-2：15%；pTR-1：38%；ORR (RECIST)：13%	1年 PFS：85%
		第2组：纳武利尤单抗×2+伊匹木单抗×1→手术	15	MPR：20%；pTR-2：33%；pTR-1：40%；ORR (RECIST)：38%	
NCT03003637 (IMCISION) Ⅱ期	Ⅱ~ⅣB 期	纳武利尤单抗×2→手术	6	MPR[c]：16%	MPR[c] 组 1 年 DFS：100%
		纳武利尤单抗×2+伊匹木单抗×1→手术	26	MPR[c]：31%	
NCT03618654 Ⅰ期	任意分期	度伐利尤单抗×1+每天二甲双胍→手术	16 HPV+；11 HPV-	PPR：60%	N/A
		度伐利尤单抗×1→手术	6 HPV+；2 HPV-	PPR：37.5%	N/A
NCT03575598 (SNOW) Ⅰ期	T2~T4aN0~N2，或 T1>1 cm N2 口腔癌	每天司曲替尼+纳武利尤单抗×1→手术	10	9/10 分期下降；1 例 pCR	中位随访超过1年未见复发
NCT03238365 Ⅰ期	任意分期	纳武利尤单抗×2±每天他达拉非→手术	47	PPR/MPR：50%；pCR：9%	N/A

（续表）

临床试验	患者入组标准	治疗方案	样本量	缓解率	复发率
NCT03342911 Ⅱ期	Ⅲ~Ⅳ期HPV−， Ⅱ~Ⅲ期HPV+	每周卡铂+紫杉醇×6+纳武利尤单抗×3→手术	26a；23 HPV−；3 HPV+	MPR: 69%, pCR: 42%； HPV−: MPR: 65%, pCR: 39%； HPV+: MPR: 100%, pCR: 67%	N/A
NCT03107182 （OPTIMA Ⅱ） Ⅱ期 TORS组	HPV+口咽癌； T1~T2扁桃体或舌根侧原发，非肿块型N2A~N2B，非下颈部淋巴结≤2个且大小≤5 cm，吸烟史≤20包	卡铂×3+每周白蛋白结合型紫杉醇×9+纳武利尤单抗×3→TORS（若影像学缓解≥50%）	9	pCR: 67%	N/A
NCT02274155 Ⅰb期	Ⅱ~ⅣA期	MEDI6469×3→手术	17	N/A	中位随访2年；PFS: 71%

HPV：人乳头瘤病毒；SCC：鳞状细胞癌；RT：放疗；CRT：化放疗；MPR：主要病理学缓解；PPR：部分病理学缓解；NPR：无病理学缓解；pTR：病理学肿瘤缓解；pCR：病理学完全缓解；PR：部分缓解；CR：完全缓解；SD：病情稳定；ORR：总缓解率；IMRT：调强放疗；TORS：经口机器人手术（transoral robotic surgery）；DFS：无病生存期；高风险：阳性切缘/包膜外扩展

a 正在招募中

b 根据RECIST标准定义缓解，但是通过将治疗前CT的测量与病理学测量进行比较

c 在试验中定义为（接近）pCR，表示残余肿瘤减少≥90%，应等同于MPR

CXCL9、CXCL10 和 CXCL11）表达均增加。

　　Wise-Draper 等（2021）开展了另一项 Ⅱ 期临床试验（NCT02641093），92 例患者在手术切除前 1~3 周接受了一定剂量的帕博利珠单抗新辅助治疗，随后再接受 6 个周期的辅助治疗；并行 60~66 Gy 的辅助性放疗，针对高风险患者则每周同步给予顺铂化疗[23-24]。该试验招募的受试者为 T3/T4 期和（或）2 个以上淋巴结受累，且大多数（88%）患者为口腔癌；在复发风险分析中 55% 的患者有高风险特征。试验主要研究终点是 1 年 DFS，与 RTOG9501 试验[25]相比较，结果显示高风险患者 1 年 DFS 为 68%（95%CI：54%~86%），与 RTOG9501 试验中的高风险患者结果（DFS 为 65%；95%CI：57%~74%）相似。而无高风险特征的患者 1 年 DFS 达 97%（95%CI：91%~100%），明显高于 RTOG9501 试验中类似患者的 DFS（69%；95%CI：59%~78%）。在这项研究中，具有主要病理学缓解或部分病理学缓解（MPR/PPR）的患者，其 1 年 DFS 达到了 100%。而对于无病理学缓解（NPR）的患者，其 1 年 DFS 则为 73%（$P=0.013$）。在这项研究中，接受治疗的患者耐受性良好，无剂量限制性毒性反应；且免疫治疗的疗效与 PD-L1 状态密切相关，PD-L1 联合阳性评分（CPS）为 0 的患者中仅有 19% 的患者获得 PPR/MPR，而 PD-L1 CPS ≥ 20% 的患者中则有 90% 的患者获得 PPR/MPR。相关研究表明，术前样本中的多个 PD-L1、PD-L2 和干扰素 γ 诱导基因与免疫治疗反应相关，包括 CXCL9、CXCL10 和 CXCL11。这与 Uppaluri 等（2020）[26]的研究数据相符，进一步证明肿瘤微环境与免疫治疗反应相关。

　　同样，有两项试验评估了术前接受纳武利尤单抗新辅助治疗的疗效，其疗程更长。Horton 等（2019）公布了一项单臂 Ⅱ 期临床试验（NCT03021993）的第一阶段结果[27]，即术前给予 3~4 周期纳武利尤单抗（双周疗法），第 4 周期需在第 3 周期治疗后根据 RECIST 标准评估肿瘤对治疗的反应或者治疗期间是否保持稳定状态来决定是否继续使用。该试验招募了 T2~T4 期的原发性口腔癌患者，主要研究终点是与组织病理学测量的肿瘤大小相比，初始肿瘤在轴向横截面上的测量总和缩小 ≥ 30%，由于影像学测量与病理学测量结果不一致，该结果有可能存在偏差。研究发现，治疗前和手术前通过 CT 扫描测量的肿瘤大小变化与病理学测量结果间存在相关性（r=0.80，P=0.014），根据该评价标准，9例患者中有4例患者对治疗有反应，其中1例患者表现为病情稳定；通过进一步分析肿瘤淋巴细胞浸润，发现疾病进展与CD4+效应记忆T细胞呈正相关，而与CD26和TIM-3呈负相关[28]。

CHECKMATE358试验是一项多队列Ⅰ/Ⅱ期临床研究，评估纳武利尤单抗新辅助治疗用于病毒相关性肿瘤[29]。HNSCC组包括T1期或以上、淋巴结阳性、可切除的患者，患者接受2周期的纳武利尤单抗新辅助治疗，随后在第2周期后的1~3周进行手术；然后按照标准程序进行辅助治疗。初步报道显示，有29例患者接受2周期的纳武利尤单抗新辅助治疗，未出现3~4级免疫相关不良事件；在23例治疗有效的患者中，50%的HPV阳性患者和46%的HPV阴性患者出现了治疗反应；有几例患者出现了疾病进展，其中1例患者的肿瘤增大了100%以上。

一些新辅助"机会窗"（window-of-opportunity, WOP）试验正在可切除的口腔癌患者中评估新的免疫检查点靶点，如OX40、TIGIT和TIM 3。OX40是一种在活化T细胞表面表达的共刺激受体，对维持免疫反应至关重要[30]。一项Ⅰb期研究评估了OX40激动剂抗体MEDI6469对患者免疫系统和肿瘤的影响，给药方式为隔天给药1次，共给药3次，最后1次给药后2天、7天或14天进行手术。共招募17例可切除的Ⅱ~ⅣA期HNSCC患者，其中11例为HPV阴性，6例为HPV阳性。中位随访时间为2年，无进展生存期为71%。在治疗过程中，有4例患者出现了免疫反应，表现为肿瘤组织和外周血中CD4+和CD8+记忆T细胞增殖增加，以及CD4+肿瘤浸润性淋巴细胞的PD-L1表达增加，这表明免疫治疗对免疫系统产生积极影响。WOP研究提供了评估生物标志物与新型药物反应机制的能力，有助于更好地理解药物的作用机制。

4　挽救性手术联合免疫治疗

局部复发性HNSCC患者的预后通常较差，为改善其预后，对围术期免疫治疗进行了专门的评估。一项单臂Ⅱ期试验（NCT03355560）评估了先前接受过明确放疗的患者在挽救性切除术后使用单药纳武利尤单抗的疗效[31]。该研究招募了39例不适合其他根治性治疗手段的患者，在术后4~11周开始接受纳武利尤单抗治疗，并持续6个月。对这些患者分析发现，其治疗耐受性良好，仅有8%的患者需要中断治疗，2年DFS为60%，明显高于以往的研究结果。

5　联合应用不同免疫治疗方式

在一项开放标签随机Ⅱ期试验中，T2~T4b期或淋巴结阳性的口腔HNSCC患者在第1周和第3周均给予纳武利尤单抗治疗，然后在第3周进行手术，第1周给予或不给予伊匹木单抗联合治疗[15]。共有14例患者被随机分配到纳武利尤单抗单药治疗组，15例患者被随机分配到纳武利尤单抗与伊匹木单抗联合治疗组。两组共同的主要终点是安全性和影像学治疗前后肿瘤体积的变化。联合治疗导致4例患者出现3级或更高的免疫相关不良事件，包括结肠炎、肺炎、关节肿胀和2次输液反应。尽管没有出现剂量限制性毒性，但由于治疗毒性、患者个人选择或对病情进展的担忧，有6例患者没有完成第2次纳武利尤单抗治疗。治疗开始后，患者进行术前影像学检查的中位时间是14天。纳武利尤单抗单药治疗组中，肿瘤体积平均缩小率50%（80%CI：31%~70%），而联合治疗组中，肿瘤体积平均缩小53%（80%CI：34%~72%）。根据RECIST标准，纳武利尤单抗单药治疗组的缓解率为13%，联合治疗组为38%。另外，纳武利尤单抗单药组治疗的病理学缓解率（pTR-1=38%，pTR-2=15%，MPR=8%）和联合治疗组的病理学缓解率（pTR-1=40%，pTR-2=33%，MPR=20%）均较显著。研究发现，PD-L1表达与治疗反应无关。多重免疫荧光显示，治疗前CD4+T细胞在总人群和接受联合治疗的亚组中可以作为预测治疗反应的标志物，而在仅接受纳武利尤单抗组的患者中则没有这种预测作用。这与NCT03021993研究[28]中提出的CD4+ T细胞的负预后价值相反。该研究还发现，在治疗前和手术后进行正电子发射计算机断层扫描（PET-CT），摄取率与治疗反应无关。

IMCISION Ⅰb/Ⅱ期临床试验评估了新辅助纳武利尤单抗单药治疗及其与伊匹木单抗联合治疗在 T2~T4 期、N0~N3 期头颈部鳞状细胞癌患者中的疗效与安全性[32]。研究共纳入 32 例患者，其中 6 例接受纳武利尤单抗单药治疗，26 例接受纳武利尤单抗联合伊匹木单抗治疗。纳武利尤单抗在术前第 1 周和第 3 周给药，伊匹木单抗在第 1 周给药，患者于第 5 周接受手术治疗。研究主要终点为病理学缓解率。结果显示，联合治疗组 31% 的患者和纳武利尤单抗单药组 16% 的患者达到"接近病理学完全缓解（near-pCR）"，定义为治疗后可存活肿瘤细胞较基线减少 ≥ 90%，基本等同于主要病理学缓解（MPR）。免疫相关不良事件方面，共有 11 例（占 32 例患者的 34%）出现 3~4 级不良反应，但均可控且可管理。PD-L1 联合阳性评分（CPS）未能有效预测治疗反应，但低氧基因表达的下降（而非基线水平）与治疗反应显著相关（$P<0.001$）[32]。

酪氨酸激酶抑制剂虽然不是免疫检查点抑制剂，但其能改变肿瘤微环境，与其他免疫治疗联合应用已在多种肿瘤中被评估。司曲替尼（sitravatinib）是一种应用前景广泛的选择性酪氨酸激酶抑制剂，在临床前模型中可使 PD-L1、PD-1 和 CTLA-4 的表达增加，并与免疫治疗产生协同效应[33]。在一项Ⅰ期 WOP 研究中，司曲替尼从第 1 天开始每天给药，第 15 天联合单剂量的纳武利尤单抗免疫治疗，于第 23~30 天进行手术[34]。该试验共招募了 10 例 T2~T4a N0~N2 期口腔癌患者；除 1 例患者外，所有患者均获得满意的病理学降期，其中 1 例患者获得病理学完全缓解。接受纳武利尤单抗治疗导致瘤内髓源性抑制细胞减少，并且在治疗反应越强的患者中越明显。目前，其他免疫治疗与酪氨酸激酶抑制剂联合使用正在复发/转移性病例中被研究，显示出有前景的疗效，但尚未在围术期病例中进行评估[35]。

二甲双胍已被证实通过改变肿瘤微环境促进抗肿瘤免疫[36]。一项随机 WOP 试验评估了度伐利尤单抗单药或与二甲双胍联合治疗的情况。在进行手术之前，35 例可切除型 HNSCC 患者接受为期 4 周的窗口期治疗；接受联合治疗的 25 例患者中，有 60% 的患者获得 PPR/MPR（病理学缓解至少达到 10%），而接受度伐利尤单抗单药治疗的 8 例患者中，PPR/MPR 仅为 37.5%。患者的治疗耐受性良好，均未出现 3 级或以上免疫或治疗相关不良事件。

一项双臂 WOP 试验将患者随机分配到纳武利尤单抗治疗组（即术前接受 2 周期纳武利尤单抗治疗）和纳武利尤单抗与他达拉非（tadalafil）联合治疗组（即在术前接受 2 周期纳武利尤单抗治疗的同时每天服用他达拉非，持续服用 4 周）。初步数据表明，使用他达拉非（磷酸二酯酶 5 抑制剂，PDE5）可能会减少 MDSC[37]。在 47 例入组患者中，观察到 75% 的患者获得了病理学缓解结果，其中 50% 的患者获得 PPR 或 MPR。这与 Wise-Draper 等报道的使用帕博利珠单抗单药治疗获得 43% 的病理学缓解结果一致[24]。根据肿瘤的转录分析结果，他达拉非治疗与肿瘤内 MDSC 浸润和 T 细胞激活增强相关。

6　化疗联合免疫治疗

化疗联合免疫治疗被认为是一种有前景的治疗策略，因为化疗会导致抗原性细胞死亡，从而增强新抗原的递呈。临床前数据还表明，不同的化疗药物可能对肿瘤微环境产生不同的影响，从而增加对免疫治疗的应答[38]。目前已有几项正在进行的试验评估了化疗与免疫治疗在新辅助治疗中的联合应用。

Zinner 等 2020 年报道了一项 Ⅱ 期临床试验，即患者每 2 周接受纳武利尤单抗新辅助治疗 3 周期，同时每周联合紫杉醇和卡铂化疗（为期 6 周），新辅助治疗完成 2 周后进行外科手术[39]。该研究入组了 4 例 Ⅱ~Ⅲ 期 HPV 阳性和 23 例 Ⅲ~Ⅳ 期 HPV 阴性的口咽部 HNSCC 患者。所有患者都完成了治疗，有 37% 的患者出现了 3~4 级毒性反应，主要与化疗相关，其中包括 4 例中性粒细胞减少症和 3 例贫血。主要研究终点是原发肿瘤的 pCR，有 26 例患者可进行评估（其中 1 例患者原发肿瘤部位不明）。HPV 阴性患者的 pCR 率和 MPR 率分别为 39% 和 65%，3 例可评估的 HPV 阳性患者的 pCR 率和 MPR 率分别为 67% 和 100%。

Rosenberg 等（2021）公布了 Ⅱ 期 OPTIMA 2 试验的初步结果，该试验评估了针对 HPV 阳性口咽癌患者进行卡铂、白蛋白结合型紫杉醇（nab-paclitaxel）和纳武利尤单抗诱导治疗 3 个周期后的反应适应性治疗[40]。有 9 例低风险患者（T1~T2 扁桃体或舌根侧原发、非肿块型 N2A~N2B、非下颈部淋巴结 ≤ 2 个且大小 ≤ 5 cm、吸烟史 ≤ 20 包年）接受了经口机器人手术（TORS）和选择性淋巴结切除术。该试验的 pCR 率（67%）与 Zinner 等（2020）[39] 的试验中 3 例 HPV 阳性患者的 pCR 率相仿。然而，患者只有对诱导化疗和免疫治疗的反应达到或超过 RECIST 标准的 50%，才有资格接受 TORS 治疗。试验结果鼓舞人心，并且与诱导化疗试验结果（如 Licitra 等 2003 年报告描述的口腔癌 pCR 率为 27%）相比，同样显示出优势，但由于该试验样本量较小，使其对围术期化疗和免疫治疗的评价受到了限制。

7　疫苗 / 细胞疗法

一些 I 期临床试验评估了疫苗用于早期辅助治疗的安全性（表 7-2）。针对 HPV 阳性 HNSCC 患者的疫苗接种试验主要将 E6/E7 蛋白作为抗原靶点。一项 I / IIa 期临床试验评估了 MEDI0457 的应用，MEDI0457 是一种编码 HPV16 和 HPV18 的 E6 和 E7 蛋白共识序列的病毒质粒，包含了重组的白介素 12（IL-12）编码剂，通过肌肉注射后使用电脉冲来辅助疫苗成分进入细胞内部[41]。该试验对疫苗的两种不同剂量进行了评估。主要研究终点是疫苗的安全性评价。试验中未发生严重不良事件，12 个月的 DFS 为 89%，有 3 例患者出现了病情进展。大多数患者的抗 HPV16/HPV18 E6/E7 反应显著增加，88% 的患者出现了

表 7-2　头颈部肿瘤围术期以疫苗为基础的试验

干预物	靶标	临床试验
HESPECTA[48]	E6	NCT02821494
MEDI-0457[41]	E6/7	NCT02163057
ADXS11-001[49]	HPV16 E7	NCT02002182
抗 MUC1 疫苗 + 他达拉非[50]	MUC1	NCT02544880
树突细胞疫苗[43]	ALDH 高表达肿瘤细胞	临床前研究
树突细胞疫苗[44]	p53	NCT00404339
树突细胞疫苗	凋亡肿瘤细胞	初步研究

抗 HPV18 E7 的血清反应。在完成疫苗接种 3 个月后，至少能检测到一种抗原的滴度。ADXS11-001（axalimogene flolisbac）是一种基于单核细胞增生症李斯特菌减毒株的重组载体疫苗，感染抗原呈递细胞并产生经过修饰的 HPV16 的 E7 蛋白，从而产生免疫反应。另外，在一项尚未公布结果的 II 期临床研究中，9 例任何分期的 HPV 阳性口咽癌患者在手术前接种了最多 2 剂疫苗，约 1/3 的患者在手术时产生了 HPV 特异性 T 细胞反应[42]。

一些研究已在 HNC 围术期测试了几种树突细胞（DC）的疫苗策略，包括针对 p53 和乙醛脱氢酶的佐剂。一项临床前研究显示，在小鼠模型中，手术切除后使用含有高表达的乙醛脱氢酶鳞状细胞癌肿瘤干细胞的 DC 疫苗接种小鼠，能够减少肿瘤局部复发，并延长宿主存活率[43]，提示可能对预防肿瘤复发和提高生存率具有潜在的治疗效果。另外一项针对 HNC 患者的基于 DC p53 肽佐剂疫苗的 I b 期临床试验[44]招募了 16 例已接受手术和辅助治疗的晚期 HNC 患者，其中 4 例患者的细胞负载了 T 辅助破伤风类毒素肽，6 例 HLA-DR4+ 患者的细胞负载了 HLA-DR4 特异性 P53 肽；3 年 DFS 为 80%，其中 3 例患者死于疾病，其余患者未复发。69% 的患者出现了 p53 肽特异性免疫反应，不同治疗组间没有显著差异。另外一项探索性研究评估了类似方案，但其使用了凋亡肿瘤细胞而不是特异性 HNSCC 抗原[45]；研究对象为已接受手术切除并完成辅助治疗的 III/IV 期 HNSCC 患者；疫苗接种通过淋巴结内注射进行，无明显毒性反应，所有患者在接种疫苗后 5 年内均未发病。

围术期这个特殊的时间点为研究以疫苗为基础的免疫疗法提供了独特机会，因为可以得到配对的术前和手术标本，从而进行有意义的相关分析。尽管目前关于围术期接种疫苗的有效性证据有限，但正在进行的试验可能会证明其价值。

8　结论

围术期免疫治疗前景可观，目前正在进行大量试验，研究各种治疗方法的影响（表 7-3）。初步数据显示，在术前使用免疫治疗可以产生治疗效果。但是免疫治疗可能需要较长的治疗时间，因此需要进行详细监测，以确保患者的安全性和疗效。虽然还需要进一步的随访，但早期结果表明，对术前免疫治疗有显著病理反应的患者表现出优异的长期生存率，与反应程度相适应的辅助治疗可为降低放疗强度并减少其相关毒性提供机会。鉴于免疫治疗在病毒介导的转移性肿瘤中取得了公认的良好疗效，免疫治疗有望成为 HPV 阳性肿瘤降期治疗的一种手段。OPTIMA Ⅱ 试验正在探索在 TORS 后用诱导化疗免疫治疗以减轻局部晚期 HPV 阳性 HNSCC 患者辅助治疗的强度。同样，NCT03715946 Ⅱ 期试验评估了降强度放疗联合纳武利尤单抗治疗术后中风险 HPV 阳性肿瘤患者的疗效。一些试验正在研究将术后免疫治疗作为一种辅助治疗策略，与放化疗联合治疗复发风险高的患者，如 NCT03480672 试验和 NIVOPOSTOP 试验。另外，随机 Ⅱ 期 PATHWay 试验正在评估帕博利珠单抗在不适合接受其他治疗的患者中的应用情况。

免疫治疗可使一些患者获得持续缓解，并且严重不良反应并不常见。生物标志物研究已经报道了临床反应与肿瘤炎症以及与干扰素 γ 相关基因特征间的相关性。然而，临床反应与 PD-L1 表达之间的相关性并不一致，并非所有 PD-L1 表达的患者都会对免疫治疗产生积极的反应。因此，需要准确的生物标志物来更好地选择接受（新）辅助免疫治疗的患者，以避免不必要的免疫相关毒性反应或延误确定性的治疗。此外，一些新型的免疫治疗间的联合应用方式以及改变肿瘤微环境的方法也正在研究中。术前免疫治疗联合放疗正在一些试验中被采用，这种治疗方式可能会因增加肿瘤炎症和新抗原形成而产生协同作用。PARP 抑制剂可上调 PD-L1 的表达，从而提高免疫治疗的疗效[46]。在围术期评估的新一代 PD-L1 抑制剂中，如结合 PD-L1 和 TGF-β 的双特异性单克隆抗体 M7824，可防止肿瘤对 PD-L1 阻断的免疫逃逸，特别是在 HPV 相关疾病中[47]。

原文符合伦理标准相关声明

Disclosure of Potential Conflicts of Interest Frederick M. Howard declares that he has no conflict of interest.

Ari Rosenberg reports advisory/consulting fees from Nanobiotix and EMD-serono.

Nishant Agrawal declares that he has no relevant conflict of interests.

表 7-3　关于头颈部鳞状细胞癌围术期免疫治疗正在进行的试验

临床试验	状态	免疫治疗药物
NCT02841748 (PATHWay)	招募中	帕博利珠单抗
NCT02769520	招募中	帕博利珠单抗
NCT04340258	尚未开始招募	帕博利珠单抗 + 铯^{131} 近距离放疗
NCT03765918 (KEYNOTE-689)	招募中	帕博利珠单抗
NCT03480672	招募中	帕博利珠单抗
NCT04323202	招募中	帕博利珠单抗
NCT03576417 (NIVOPOSTOP)	招募中	纳武利尤单抗
NCT03700905 (IMSTAR-HN)	活跃，未招募	纳武利尤单抗 ± 伊匹木单抗
NCT04169074	招募中	纳武利尤单抗 + 阿贝西利
NCT03878979	招募中	纳武利尤单抗
NCT03247712	活跃，未招募	纳武利尤单抗 + 放疗
NCT03906526	招募中	纳武利尤单抗 +VTX-2337
NCT03854032	招募中	纳武利尤单抗 +BMS986205
NCT03721757 (NICO)	活跃，未招募	纳武利尤单抗
NCT03715946	活跃，未招募	纳武利尤单抗
NCT03406247 (ADJORL1)	尚未开始招募	纳武利尤单抗 + 伊匹木单抗
NCT03635164	活跃，未招募	度伐利尤单抗 + 放疗
NCT03737968	招募中	度伐利尤单抗 ± 替西木单抗
NCT03174275	招募中	度伐利尤单抗
NCT03529422	招募中	度伐利尤单抗 + 放疗
NCT02827838	招募中	度伐利尤单抗
NCT03618134	招募中	立体定向放疗 + 度伐利尤单抗 ± 替西木单抗
NCT04116047 (CompARE)	招募中	度伐利尤单抗
NCT01810913	招募中	阿替利珠单抗
NCT03708224	活跃，未招募	阿替利珠单抗 ± 托珠单抗（tocilizumab）
NCT03452137	招募中	阿替利珠单抗
NCT03336606	活跃，未招募	MEDI0562
NCT04247282	已暂停	M7824 ± TriAd 疫苗
NCT03821272	招募中	PepCan 疫苗
NCT04166006	招募中	树突细胞疫苗
NCT03552718	状态未知	新抗原酵母疫苗

参考文献

1. O'Sullivan B, Huang SH, Su J et al (2016) Development and validation of a staging system for HPV-related oropharyngeal cancer by the International Collaboration on Oropharyngeal cancer Network for Staging (ICON-S): a multicentre cohort study. Lancet Oncol 17:440-451. https://doi.org/10.1016/S1470-2045(15)00560-4
2. Iyer NG, Tan DSW, Tan VKM et al (2015) Randomized trial comparing surgery and adjuvant radiotherapy versus concurrent chemoradiotherapy in patients with advanced, nonmetastatic squamous cell carcinoma of the head and neck: 10-year update and subset analysis. Cancer 121:1599-1607. https://doi.org/10.1002/cncr.29251
3. Stenson KM, Kunnavakkam R, Cohen EEW et al (2010) Chemoradiation for patients with advanced oral cavity cancer. Laryngoscope 120:93-99. https://doi.org/10.1002/lary.20716
4. Licitra L, Grandi C, Guzzo M et al (2003) Primary chemotherapy in resectable oral cavity squamous cell cancer: a randomized controlled trial. J Clin Oncol 21:327-333. https://doi.org/10.1200/JCO.2003.06.146
5. Department of Veterans Affairs Laryngeal Cancer Study Group, Wolf GT, Fisher SG et al (1991) Induction chemotherapy plus radiation compared with surgery plus radiation in patients with advanced laryngeal cancer. N Engl J Med 324:1685-1690. https://doi.org/10.1056/NEJM199106133242402
6. Seiwert TY, Foster CC, Blair EA et al (2019) OPTIMA: a phase II dose and volume de-escalation trial for human papillomavirus-positive oropharyngeal cancer. Ann Oncol 30:297-302. https://doi.org/10.1093/annonc/mdy522
7. Cohen EEW, Karrison TG, Kocherginsky M et al (2014) Phase III randomized trial of induction chemotherapy in patients with N2 or N3 locally advanced head and neck cancer. J Clin Oncol 32:2735-2743. https://doi.org/10.1200/JCO.2013.54.6309
8. Colevas AD, Busse PM, Norris CM et al (1998) Induction chemotherapy with docetaxel, cisplatin, fluorouracil, and leucovorin for squamous cell carcinoma of the head and neck: a phase I/II trial. J Clin Oncol. https://doi.org/10.1200/JCO.1998.16.4.1331
9. Kwiatkowski DJ, Rusch VW, Chaft JE et al (2019) Neoadjuvant atezolizumab in resectable non-small cell lung cancer (NSCLC): interim analysis and biomarker data from a multicenter study (LCMC3). J Clin Oncol. https://doi.org/10.1200/JCO.2019.37.15_suppl.8503
10. Forde PM, Spicer J, Lu S et al (2021) Abstract CT003: Nivolumab (NIVO) + platinum-doublet chemotherapy (chemo) vs chemo as neoadjuvant treatment (tx) for resectable (IB-IIIA) non-small cell lung cancer (NSCLC) in the phase 3 CheckMate 816 trial. Cancer Res. https://doi.org/10.1158/1538-7445. AM2021-CT003
11. Howard FM, Villamar D, He G et al (2021) The emerging role of immune checkpoint inhibitors for the treatment of breast cancer. Expert Opin Investig Drugs. https://doi.org/10.1080/13543784.2022.1986002
12. Spaulding MB, Fischer SG, Wolf GT (1994) Tumor response, toxicity, and survival after neoadjuvant organ-preserving chemotherapy for advanced laryngeal carcinoma. The Department of Veterans Affairs Cooperative Laryngeal Cancer Study Group. J Clin Oncol 12:1592-1599. https://doi.org/10.1200/JCO.1994.12.8.1592
13. Hellmann MD, Chaft JE, William WN et al (2014) Pathologic response after neoadjuvant

chemotherapy in resectable non-small cell lung cancers: proposal for the use of "major pathologic response" as a surrogate endpoint. Lancet Oncol 15:e42-e50. https://doi.org/10.1016/S1470-2045(13)70334-6
14. Cottrell TR, Thompson ED, Forde PM et al (2018) Pathologic features of response to neoadjuvant anti-PD-1 in resected non-small-cell lung carcinoma: a proposal for quantitative immune-related pathologic response criteria (irPRC). Ann Oncol 29:1853-1860. https://doi.org/10.1093/annonc/mdy218
15. Schoenfeld JD, Hanna GJ, Jo VY et al (2020) Neoadjuvant nivolumab or nivolumab plus ipilimumab in untreated oral cavity squamous cell carcinoma: a phase 2 open-label randomized clinical trial. JAMA Oncol 6:1563-1570. https://doi.org/10.1001/jamaoncol.2020.2955
16. Uppaluri R, Campbell KM, Egloff AM et al (2020) Neoadjuvant and adjuvant pembrolizumab in resectable locally advanced, human papillomavirus-unrelated head and neck cancer: a multicenter, phase II trial. Clin Cancer Res 26:5140-5152. https://doi.org/10.1158/1078-0432.CCR-20-1695
17. Patil V, Noronha V, Joshi A et al (2013) Is there a limitation of RECIST criteria in prediction of pathological response, in head and neck cancers, to postinduction chemotherapy? ISRN Oncol. https://doi.org/10.1155/2013/259154
18. Baghi M, Mack MG, Hambek M et al (2007) Usefulness of MRI volumetric evaluation in patients with squamous cell cancer of the head and neck treated with neoadjuvant chemotherapy. Head Neck 29:104-108. https://doi.org/10.1002/hed.20488
19. Lauber K, Dunn L (2019) Immunotherapy mythbusters in head and neck cancer: the abscopal effect and pseudoprogression. Am Soc Clin Oncol Educ Book 39:352-363. https://doi.org/10.1200/EDBK_238339
20. Ferris RL, Blumenschein G, Fayette J et al (2016) Nivolumab for recurrent squamous-cell carcinoma of the head and neck. N Engl J Med. https://doi.org/10.1056/NEJMoa1602252
21. Rosenberg AJ, Agrawal N, Pearson A et al (2020) Low risk HPV associated oropharyngeal squamous cell carcinoma treated with induction chemoimmunotherapy followed by TORS or radiotherapy. Int J Radiat Oncol Biol Phys 106:1123. https://doi.org/10.1016/j.ijrobp.2019.11.342
22. Bernier J, Domenge C, Ozsahin M et al (2004) Postoperative irradiation with or without concomitant chemotherapy for locally advanced head and neck cancer. N Engl J Med 350:1945-1952. https://doi.org/10.1056/NEJMoa032641
23. Wise-Draper T, Gulati S, Takiar V et al (2020) 809 Phase 2 trial of neoadjuvant and adjuvant PD-1 checkpoint blockade in local-regionally advanced, resectable HNSCC indicates pathological response is associated with high disease-free survival. J Immunother Cancer. https://doi.org/10.1136/jitc-2020-SITC2020.0809
24. Wise-Draper TM, Takiar V, Mierzwa ML et al (2021) Association of pathological response to neoadjuvant pembrolizumab with tumor PD-L1 expression and high disease-free survival (DFS) in patients with resectable, local-regionally advanced, head and neck squamous cell carcinoma (HNSCC). J Clin Oncol. https://doi.org/10.1200/JCO.2021.39.15_suppl.6006
25. Cooper JS, Pajak TF, Forastiere AA et al (2004) Postoperative concurrent radiotherapy and chemotherapy for high-risk squamous-cell carcinoma of the head and neck. N Engl J Med 350:1937-1944. https://doi.org/10.1056/NEJMoa032646
26. Kim E, Palackdharry S, Yaniv B et al (2018) Gene expression signature after one dose of neoadjuvant pembrolizumab associated with tumor response in head and neck squamous cell carcinoma (HNSCC). J Clin Oncol. https://doi.org/10.1200/JCO.2018.36.15_suppl.6059

27. Horton JD, Knochelmann H, Armeson K et al (2019) Neoadjuvant presurgical PD-1 inhibition in oral cavity squamous cell carcinoma. J Clin Oncol. https://doi.org/10.1200/JCO.2019.37.15_suppl.2574
28. Knochelmann H, Horton JD, Meek M et al (2019) Immune signatures associated with response to neoadjuvant PD-1 blockade in oral cavity cancer. J Clin Oncol. https://doi.org/10.1200/JCO.2019.37.15_suppl.6055
29. Ferris RL, Gonçalves A, Baxi SS et al (2017) An open-label, multicohort, phase 1/2 study in patients with virus-associated cancers (CheckMate 358): safety and efficacy of neoadjuvant nivolumab in squamous cell carcinoma of the head and neck (SCCHN). Ann Oncol 28:v628-v629. https://doi.org/10.1093/annonc/mdx440.041
30. Aspeslagh S, Postel-Vinay S, Rusakiewicz S et al (2016) Rationale for anti-OX40 cancer immunotherapy. Eur J Cancer 52:50-66. https://doi.org/10.1016/j.ejca.2015.08.021
31. Leddon J, Haque S, Gulati S et al (2021) Adjuvant nivolumab following salvage resection in head and neck squamous cell carcinoma patients previously treated with definitive therapy: a single-arm phase II multi-institutional study. J Clin Oncol. https://doi.org/10.1200/JCO.2021.39.15_suppl.6031
32. Zuur L, Vos JL, Elbers JB et al (2020) LBA40 Neoadjuvant nivolumab and nivolumab plus ipilimumab induce (near-) complete responses in patients with head and neck squamous cell carcinoma: the IMCISION trial. Ann Oncol 31:S1169. https://doi.org/10.1016/j.annonc.2020.08.2270
33. Du W, Huang H, Sorrelle N, Brekken RA Sitravatinib potentiates immune checkpoint blockade in refractory cancer models. JCI Insight. https://doi.org/10.1172/jci.insight.124184
34. Bernal MO, Araujo DV, Chepeha DB et al (2020) SNOW: sitravatinib and nivolumab in oral cavity cancer (OCC) window of opportunity study. J Clin Oncol. https://doi.org/10.1200/JCO.2020.38.15_suppl.6569
35. Chen TH, Chang PMH, Yang MH (2021) Combination of pembrolizumab and lenvatinib is a potential treatment option for heavily pre-treated recurrent and metastatic head and neck cancer. J Chin Med Assoc 84:361-367. https://doi.org/10.1097/JCMA.0000000000000497
36. Kurelac I, Umesh Ganesh N, Iorio M et al (2020) The multifaceted effects of metformin on tumor microenvironment. Semin Cell Dev Biol 98:90-97. https://doi.org/10.1016/j.semcdb.2019.05.010
37. Luginbuhl AJ, Johnson JM, Harshyne L et al (2019) A window of opportunity trial of preoperative nivolumab with or without tadalafil in squamous cell carcinoma of the head and neck (SCCHN): safety, clinical, and correlative outcomes. Ann Oncol. https://doi.org/10.1093/annonc/mdz252.008
38. Zitvogel L, Apetoh L, Ghiringhelli F et al (2008) Immunological aspects of cancer chemotherapy. Nat Rev Immunol 8:59-73. https://doi.org/10.1038/nri2216
39. Zinner R, Johnson JM, Tuluc M et al (2020) Neoadjuvant nivolumab (N) plus weekly carboplatin (C) and paclitaxel (P) in resectable locally advanced head and neck cancer. J Clin Oncol. https://doi.org/10.1200/JCO.2020.38.15_suppl.6583
40. Rosenberg A, Agrawal N, Pearson AT et al (2021) Nivolumab, nabpaclitaxel, and carboplatin followed by risk/response adaptive de-escalated locoregional therapy for HPV-associated oropharyngeal cancer: OPTIMA II trial. J Clin Oncol. https://doi.org/10.1200/JCO.2021.39.15_suppl.6011
41. Aggarwal C, Cohen RB, Morrow MP et al (2019) Immunotherapy targeting HPV 16/18 generates potent immune responses in HPV-associated head and neck cancer. Clin Cancer Res 25:110-124.

https://doi.org/10.1158/1078-0432. CCR-18-1763
42. Sikora A (2020) Window of opportunity trial of neoadjuvant ADXS 11-001 vaccination prior to robot-assisted resection of HPV-positive oropharyngeal squamous cell carcinoma. https://clinicaltrials.gov. Accessed 2 Jul 2021
43. Hu Y, Lu L, Xia Y et al (2016) Therapeutic efficacy of cancer stem cell vaccines in the adjuvant setting. Cancer Res 76:4661-4672. https://doi.org/10.1158/0008-5472. CAN-15-2664
44. Schuler PJ, Harasymczuk M, Visus C et al (2014) Phase I dendritic cell p53 peptide vaccine for head and neck cancer. Clin Cancer Res 20:2433-2444. https://doi.org/10.1158/1078-0432. CCR-13-2617
45. Whiteside TL, Ferris RL, Szczepanski M et al (2016) Dendritic cell-based autologous tumor vaccines for head and neck squamous cell carcinoma: promise vs reality. Head Neck 38:E494-E501. https://doi.org/10.1002/hed.24025
46. Jiao S, Xia W, Yamaguchi H et al (2017) PARP inhibitor upregulates PD-L1 expression and enhances cancer-associated immunosuppression. Clin Cancer Res 23:3711-3720. https://doi.org/10.1158/1078-0432. CCR-16-3215
47. Knudson KM, Hicks KC, Luo X et al (2018) M7824, a novel bifunctional anti-PD-L1/TGFβ trap fusion protein, promotes anti-tumor efficacy as monotherapy and in combination with vaccine. Onco Targets Ther. https://doi.org/10.1080/2162402X.2018.1426519
48. Slingerland M, Speetjens F, Welters M et al (2016) A phase I study in patients with a human papillomavirus type 16 positive oropharyngeal tumor treated with second generation synthetic long peptide vaccine conjugated to a defined adjuvant. J Clin Oncol. https://doi.org/10.1200/JCO.2016.34.15_suppl.TPS3113
49. Miles BA, Monk BJ, Safran HP (2017) Mechanistic insights into ADXS11-001 human papillomavirus-associated cancer immunotherapy. Gynecol Oncol Res Pract. https://doi.org/10.1186/s40661-017-0046-9
50. Weed DT, Zilio S, Reis IM et al (2019) The reversal of immune exclusion mediated by tadalafil and an anti-tumor vaccine also induces PDL1 upregulation in recurrent head and neck squamous cell carcinoma: interim analysis of a phase I clinical trial. Front Immunol. https://doi.org/10.3389/fimmu.2019.01206

第8章 免疫检查点抑制剂在罕见头颈部肿瘤治疗中的作用

The Role of Immune Checkpoint Inhibitors in the Treatment of Less Common Head and Neck Cancers

（Stefano Cavalieri, Paolo Bossi, Lisa Licitra 著）

（周亚娟，余笑言，鲁瑛 译）

摘要

免疫检查点抑制剂在罕见头颈部肿瘤（包括非鳞状细胞癌）中的作用尚不明确。本章将重点介绍免疫治疗在唾液腺癌（salivary gland carcinoma, SGC）和鼻腔鼻窦癌（paranasal sinus carcinomas, PNC）中的现有研究数据。

在 SGC 中，一些高级别非腺样囊性癌具有免疫活化的微环境，因此可能从免疫治疗中获益。相反，由于腺样囊性癌（adenoid cystic carcinoma, ACC）有类似免疫沙漠的微环境，免疫治疗较少产生临床获益。理论上与其他靶向治疗（如雄激素受体阳性唾液腺导管癌的雄激素剥夺疗法）的联

原作者信息

S. Cavalieri · L. Licitra (✉)
Head and Neck Medical Oncology Department, Fondazione IRCCS Istituto Nazionale dei Tumori, Milan, Italy

Department of Oncology and Hemato-Oncology, University of Milan, Milan, Italy
e-mail: stefano.cavalieri@istitutotumori.mi.it; lisa.licitra@istitutotumori.mi.it

P. Bossi
Medical Oncology Department, University of Brescia, Brescia, Italy
e-mail: paolo.bossi@unibs.it

合可能增加免疫检查点抑制剂的疗效，但仍需要进一步的研究。

与常见的 HNSCC 类似，PNC 的组织学类型通常为鳞状细胞癌，可能对免疫检查点抑制剂产生反应。鼻窦未分化癌（sinonasal undifferentiated carcinoma, SNUC）可能受益于免疫治疗，应设计对局部晚期 SNUC 进行诱导化疗的临床研究。肠型腺癌（intestinal-type adenocarcinoma, ITAC）具有类似免疫沙漠的微环境，可能难以从免疫治疗中获益。对于 SGC 和 PNC，免疫治疗并非标准治疗，因此不应在临床试验之外实施。

关键词

腺样囊性癌·肠型腺癌·非腺样囊性癌·NUT 癌（中线癌）·鼻腔鼻窦癌·唾液腺癌·鼻窦癌·鼻窦未分化癌

1 引言

无论是作为一线治疗还是作为铂类耐药的二线治疗，抗 PD-1 药物的引入已然改变了复发 / 转移性头颈鳞状细胞癌的治疗格局[1]。相比之下，在包括非鳞状细胞癌（non-SCC）在内的罕见头颈部肿瘤中，免疫检查点抑制剂的作用尚不清楚。本章将重点介绍免疫治疗在唾液腺癌和鼻窦癌中的现有研究数据。

2 唾液腺癌

唾液腺癌（SGC）是一类具有异质性的腺癌，已鉴定出 20 多种组织学亚型[2]。SGC 可能来自大唾液腺和小唾液腺。大唾液腺包括腮腺、颌下腺和舌下腺，而小唾液腺癌可存在于上呼吸消化道的任何区域，包括鼻旁窦。

SGC 相当少见。2003—2007 年，欧洲 SGC 的年龄调整发病率为 1.135/100 000 人年（95%CI：1.113~1.158），估计欧洲每年有 7838 例

新病例[3]。在临床可行的情况下，根治性手术切除是 SGC 的主要治疗手段。放射治疗，无论是传统的光子还是强子（尤其是质子或碳离子），都可作为不可切除肿瘤或术后的主要治疗手段，特别是在局部复发风险高的情况下，如腺样囊性癌、高级别肿瘤、切缘阳性、淋巴血管和（或）神经周围浸润、局部晚期[4]。

全身治疗的作用，尤其是与放疗同步时的作用，仍然需要在临床实践中得到进一步验证，相关临床试验正在进行中[4]。

复发/转移性唾液腺癌（R/M SGC）的治疗以全身治疗为主，治疗方案的选择主要基于组织学亚型[5]。对于雄激素受体（androgen receptor, AR）过度表达的亚型，患者可以接受类似于前列腺癌的内分泌治疗。同时也有 II 期研究结果表明，抗 HER2 治疗可能对表达人表皮生长因子受体 2（human epidermal growth factor receptor 2, HER2）受体的 SGC 有效[6]。

SGC 可能存在多种突变[7]，在某些情况下，这些突变可能是特定抑制剂（例如 BRAF、RET 抑制剂）的靶点[8]。鉴于临床上 R/M SGC 尚缺乏理想的治疗手段，寻找适合靶向治疗的突变靶点是一种合理的尝试。此外，欧洲肿瘤内科学会（European Society for Medical Oncology, ESMO）支持对 SGC 中的肿瘤突变负荷（TMB）进行分析[9]。值得注意的是，SGC 的发病率在乳腺癌基因（BRCA）阳性的家族中较高[10]，从而使这部分 ACC 也许能够参考乳腺癌进行临床研究及相应的靶向治疗。此外，SGC 的肿瘤微环境（TME）与在 HNSCC 中观察到的不同，尤其是在 PD-L1 阳性率方面。总体而言，存在 PD-L1 或 PD-L2 表达，或存在 PD-L1/PD-L2 共表达的 SGC 组织学亚型与较差的预后相关，无论肿瘤浸润性淋巴细胞（TIL）表达高或表达低皆如此[11]。此外，有证据表明不同组织学亚型的免疫 TME 存在差异[12]。ACC 具有类似免疫沙漠的 TME，TMB 较低，与气管 ACC 类似[13]。而唾液管癌（SDC）通常具有较高的 TMB 并表现出明显的免疫浸润[12]。BRCA1/BRCA2 突变在 DNA 修复中具有重要作用，通常与较高的 TMB 相关，因此种系 BRCA 突变中产生的 SGC 可能从免疫治疗中获益[14-15]。鉴于这些差异，下面将对目前已有免疫治疗相关数据的 SGC 类型分别进行介绍。目前通常根据临床治疗和生物学行为的不同将 SGC 分为 ACC 和 non-ACC。

2.1 腺样囊性癌

在形态学上，腺样囊性癌（ACC）是一种由导管细胞和肌上皮细胞组成的双相分化肿瘤，其特征是不同程度的实性、管状和筛状形态[16]。在临床中，ACC 可能既存在局部浸润的生物学行为，又有远处转移的倾向。

ACC 的一些临床和病理因素已被证实与预后相关。在 R/M ACC 中，转移部位、性别和无疾病间隔时间被证明是独立的预后因素[17]。对于寡转移灶的 ACC 患者，局部治疗可能带来获益，如肺转移瘤切除术或肝局部消融[4]。当需要全身治疗时，目前最有效的手段是多靶点酪氨酸激酶抑制剂，例如乐伐替尼或阿西替尼，但顺铂和蒽环类药物化疗对一小部分 ACC 患者也可能有效[5]。

此外，ACC 在 SGC 中具有独特的分子特征。大多数 ACC 具有 MYB、MYBL1 或 NFIB 基因融合[18]。这些基因突变有助于 ACC 的鉴别诊断，但没有预后意义[19]。在 ACC 中 13% 的病例检测到 NOTCH1 基因突变[7]。存在 NOTCH1 突变的 ACC 预后较差，并且容易发生肝转移和骨转移[20]。

ACC 的基因组异质性伴随着较低的体细胞突变率[7]。最近的基因组研究表明 ACC 可被分为两种分子亚型：① ACC-Ⅰ型：由 MYC 信号通过 NOTCH 突变或直接扩增驱动，进而抑制 p63 信号转导；② ACC-Ⅱ型：由 p63 驱动表皮生长因子受体（EGFR）或其他受体酪氨酸激酶来促进增殖[21]。

ACC 具有类似免疫沙漠的 TME，TIL 浸润水平较低，并且缺乏 PD-L1 表达[11, 22-23]。而免疫抑制分子 PD-L2 则在大多数（原发灶：60%；远处转移灶：73%）ACC 中表达[22]。这一发现和人类白细胞抗原 HLA-G（一种肿瘤免疫耐受的生物标志物）在 ACC 中的过度表达证实了该类型肿瘤存在免疫逃逸[23]。

一系列小样本研究已证实抗 PD-1 治疗在 ACC 中具有一定效果[24]。然而，在回顾性研究[25]和临床试验中观察到的客观缓解率（ORR）总体上并不尽如人意。在一项Ⅱ期临床试验中，帕博利珠单抗联合组蛋白脱乙酰酶抑制剂（HDAC）伏立诺他治疗 HNSCC 和 SGC 患者的 ORR 为 8%（1/12）[26]。2019 年，法国研究者公布了纳武利尤单抗治疗 R/M

SGC 的 II 期 NISCAHN 研究的初步结果 [27]。在 ACC 队列中，ORR 为 8.7%（4/46）。在一项探索伊匹木单抗联合纳武利尤单抗联合治疗 ACC 的 II 期研究中，ORR 仅为 6%（2/32）[28]。在另一项使用同样药物组合的 SWOG S1609 DART 研究中，ACC 队列中的 ORR 为 4%（1/26）[29]。尽管在 Ib 期 KEYNOTE-028 研究中，接受帕博利珠单抗治疗的 2 例 R/M ACC 患者里有 1 例观察到轻微的肿瘤缩小，但没有观察到客观缓解 [30]。另一项纳入 10 例 R/M ACC 患者的随机对照 II 期研究中，无论在接受帕博利珠单抗的同时联合或不联合姑息性放疗，均未能观察到照射野外的反应 [31]。

总之，ACC 免疫疗法进一步发展的唯一机会可能是与靶向治疗联合使用。目前有阿西替尼联合 PD-L1 抗体阿维鲁单抗 [32] 以及乐伐替尼联合帕博利珠单抗 [33] 的两项临床研究正在积极招募 ACC 患者。

2.2 非腺样囊性癌

非腺样囊性癌（non-ACC）是一类具有异质性的 SGC，包括 20 多种组织学亚型 [2, 16]。直到最近几年，R/M non-ACC 的全身治疗方法一直是铂类联合蒽环类或紫杉类药物的化疗 [34]。一些 non-ACC 的突变可能具有特征性（如分泌性癌中 ETV6 易位常伴有 NTRK3 突变 [35]），也有一些突变可作为常见的标记物（如 SDC 中的 AR[16]）。因此，在正确的临床和病理背景下进行分子学评估可能为 R/M non-ACC 的个体化治疗带来更多选择。例如，雄激素剥夺治疗用于 AR 阳性的 SDC[36]，以及抗 HER2 药物用于 HER2 扩增的 SGC 均表现出良好的临床效果，特别是曲妥珠单抗 [6]、恩美曲妥珠单抗 [37] 和德曲妥珠单抗 [38]。MyPathway 研究是一项基于分子表达谱分析的 IIa 期临床试验，评估靶向治疗在 R/M SGC 中的疗效。该研究 63% 的病例获得了客观缓解，主要与抗 HER2 药物有关 [8]。

如前所述，non-ACC 中 TME 的免疫激活程度较 ACC 更高。58% 的 non-ACC 表达 PD-L1，并且在超过一半的病例中观察到显著的免疫浸润 [11]。此外，ACC 与 non-ACC 具有相似的 PD-L2 表达水平（ACC：45%；non-ACC：32%）[11]。

不同于 ACC，部分 non-ACC 患者中观察到了免疫治疗的临床获益。

MyPathway 研究报道了 1 例黏液表皮样癌（唯一一种具有高 TMB 的 SGC 类型）患者用阿替利珠单抗作为一线治疗，实现部分缓解[8]。在帕博利珠单抗加伏立诺他的Ⅱ期临床试验中，non-ACC 患者的 ORR 为 23%（3/13）[26]，其中 2 例腺泡细胞癌患者和 1 例淋巴上皮癌患者观察到 PR。

在Ⅰb 期 KEYNOTE-028 研究的 SGC 队列中，整个 SGC 人群的 ORR 为 12%（2 例 ACC 和 24 例 non-ACC）。在 non-ACC 人群中，观察到 3 例 PR：2 例腺癌和 1 例"高级别浆液性癌"[30]。浆液性癌不包括在 WHO 2017 年分类中[2]，故我们假设其可能指腺泡细胞癌，因为腺泡细胞癌具有典型的浆液性腺泡分化[16]。

在 NISCAHN Ⅱ期临床试验的 non-ACC 队列中，ORR 为 3.8%（2/52）[27]。一项Ⅱ期临床研究使用伊匹木单抗联合纳武利尤单抗治疗 32 例 non-ACC SGC 患者，初步结果显示在 5 例患者中观察到 PR（ORR 16%）[39]，包括 3 例涎腺导管癌、1 例 AR+ve 高级别癌（可能是非特异性腺癌，NOS）以及 1 例肌上皮癌。在其余 non-ACC 组织学亚型中未观察到客观缓解，包括腺泡细胞癌、多形性腺瘤和分泌性癌。另一项类似研究的初步结果显示伊匹木单抗联合纳武利尤单抗治疗 non-ACC 患者的 ORR 较低（9%，3/35）[29]。

作为关于 SGC 免疫治疗的一般性声明，美国临床肿瘤学会（ASCO）2021 年指南建议"目前不应常规应用免疫检查点抑制剂，除非对于有特定分子改变（高 TMB、MSI-H）的患者"。然而，该小组成员称这一声明是基于非正式共识，由于证据水平较低，推荐力度较弱。系列回顾性研究表明，10%~14% 的 non-ACC 中可观察到高 TMB，并且在分析的 30 例 SGC 中没有检测到 MSI[11]。

基于目前的情况，我们主张根据欧洲肿瘤内科学会（ESMO）指南检测 non-ACC SGC 的 TMB，有助于筛选患者参加免疫治疗的临床试验。此外，目前也亟待开发增强 TME 免疫反应的新方法。对于已应用多种基于组织学的循证治疗手段，但仍治疗失败的患者，在权衡潜在风险和潜在获益后，应在临床试验中提供免疫治疗选择。因此，建议在 R/M SGC 患者的管理中施行规范的多学科诊疗，并邀请病理学专家参与。

3　鼻腔鼻窦癌

鼻腔鼻窦癌（即鼻腔和鼻窦发生的恶性肿瘤，PNC）较为少见，病理类型包括肉瘤、黑色素瘤和恶性淋巴瘤。2003—2007年，欧洲鼻窦上皮癌的年龄调整发病率为0.368/100 000人年（95%CI：0.355~0.381），估算欧洲每年新发病例为2564例[3]。

在鼻窦癌（sinonasal carcinoma, SNC）中，WHO分类第4版定义了至少六种病理类型：鳞状细胞癌（SCC）——包括三种主要亚型（角化性癌、非角化性癌、梭形细胞癌）、鼻窦未分化癌（SNUC）、淋巴上皮癌、NUT癌（中线癌）、神经内分泌癌及其小细胞和大细胞变异、肠型腺癌和非肠型腺癌[2]。最近，SMARCB1缺失的SNUC/SCC已被确定为新的病理亚型，比表达SMARCB1的亚型更具侵袭性[40]。2013年确定的另一个病理类型是具有腺样囊性特征的人乳头瘤病毒（HPV）相关性癌[41]。最近，这种亚型被重新命名为HPV相关的多表型鼻窦癌[42]。新定义的病理类型使鼻窦癌的分类变得更加复杂，需要随着时间的推移不断更新。

局部和局部区域晚期SNC采用多模式综合治疗。目前，免疫治疗在局部晚期SNC中疗效不佳，而诱导化疗在SNUC中显示出临床获益[43]。因此，局部晚期SNUC的治疗方案应在诱导化疗的基础上根据客观反应进行调整。尽管临床研究很少，但这一思路也同样适用于其他组织学亚型，因为诱导化疗在鼻窦神经内分泌癌、SCC和TP53野生型ITAC中均有明显疗效，并可能有利于降低局部复发率和远处转移率。在诱导或姑息治疗中，最常用以顺铂为基础的化疗方案，如顺铂与依托泊苷联合用于SNEC、顺铂与5-FU及亚叶酸联合用于ITAC、顺铂与5-FU及多西他赛联合用于SCC和SNUC。目前对于不适合局部治疗的R/M SNC，主要治疗方法是化疗，此种情况下患者预后很差。SNC缺乏可用的靶向治疗靶点，目前被报道的仅有非ITAC中的ETV6基因重排[42]、转化自内翻性乳头状瘤的鼻腔SCC的EGFR突变[44]以及SNUC中的IDH-2突变[45]等。

PNC具有独特的发生过程和组织学异质性，与其他更为常见的HNSCC不同，所以PNC尚未被纳入重要的一线和二线免疫治疗研究中[46-48]。美国食品药品监督管理局（FDA）和欧洲药品管理局（EMA）批准的 R/M 头颈部肿瘤一线和二线免疫治疗仅限于 SCC，没有具体提及 SNC。然而，美国国家综合癌症网络（NCCN）指南建议，筛窦和上颌窦的 R/M SCC 应遵循与 HNSCC 相同的治疗流程。迄今唯一公开招募 SNC 患者的免疫治疗临床试验是一项关于帕博利珠单抗联合西妥昔单抗疗效的 II 期研究[49]，目前免疫治疗在 R/M SNC 中的疗效报道仅限于病例报告[50]。

3.1 鼻窦鳞状细胞癌

鼻窦鳞状细胞癌的免疫特征与在 HNSCC 中观察到的一致。其中大多数（88%）具有 CD8+ TIL，其中 19% 为高表达（CD8+ TIL＞10%）。在这部分肿瘤中，PD-L1＞5% 常与 CD8+ TIL 共表达[51]。在 26% 的 SCC 中观察到 TPS ＞50%（18 例 PD-L1 阳性病例中的 14 例，共分析 54 例 SCC）[52]。这与临床研究中一线和二线应用帕博利珠单抗治疗 R/M HNSCC 的结果一致（分别为 22% 和 26%）[47-48]。仅 PD-L1 无法作为鼻窦癌的预后生物标志物[52]，但其与 CD8+ TIL 的共表达与 SCC 的较差预后相关[51]。由于这一类肿瘤具有一定的免疫原性，因此和 HNSCC 类似，PD-L1 高表达可能可以预测鼻腔 SCC 免疫治疗的获益。

3.2 鼻窦未分化癌

高级别 SNC 的基因表达分析显示，以下三组癌中的每一组都具有独特的免疫特征：①鼻窦未分化癌（SNUC）和 SMARCB1 缺失型癌；②神经内分泌癌；③包括畸胎癌肉瘤、腺癌和 NUT 癌在内的高级别癌，这三组中的每一组都具有独特的免疫特征[53]。进一步的基因表达研究表明，SNUC 的特点是免疫成分的表达，如 CD8+ 效应记忆细胞、RGS1 的调控因子（RGS1 是一种参与趋化因子信号转导调节的分子）[54]。尽管 SNUC 患者从未被纳入免疫治疗的临床试验，但已有一些抗 PD-1 治疗在 SNUC 中产生显著疗效的病例报告[50]。

3.3 肠型鼻窦腺癌

肠型鼻窦腺癌是一种腺上皮恶性肿瘤，在木材和皮革工人中发病率相对较高[2]。标准治疗是手术及术后放疗，而顺铂+5-FU+亚叶酸钙（PFL方案）化疗可使40%的患者获得病理学完全缓解。在具有野生型或功能性TP53的ITAC中，这一比例明显高于TP53突变或表达受损p53蛋白的肿瘤。因此，TP53表达的评估可能有助于指导ITAC的管理[55]。目前，没有证据表明免疫治疗可用于ITAC。在欧洲一项针对133例ITAC患者的研究中，57%的肿瘤表达低TIL，26%表达PD-L1[56]。另一个研究也得到了相似的结果，该研究报道126例ITAC中有17%表达PD-L1[52]。目前没有观察到以上两种生物标志物在ITAC中的预后作用。

3.4 嗅神经母细胞瘤

嗅神经母细胞瘤（esthesioneuroblastoma，ENB）是一种颅底神经外胚层恶性肿瘤，常发生于上鼻腔[2]。高级别肿瘤（Hyams分类Ⅲ级和Ⅳ级）的预后比Ⅰ~Ⅱ级更差。目前尚缺乏ENB免疫治疗的临床数据。在ENB中探索性使用免疫检查点抑制剂，至少在HyamsⅢ~Ⅳ级病例中可能是合理的，因为一项小型回顾性分析发现ENB原发灶中10例有4例表达PD-L1，转移灶中4例有3例表达PD-L1[57]。在同一项研究中，PD-L1阳性ENB的CD8+ TIL明显高于PD-L1阴性病例。然而，对14例患者进行的另一项回顾性研究显示ENB的TMB较低[57]。因此，应在临床试验中对ENB免疫治疗的疗效进行评估。

3.5 NUT癌（中线癌）

NUT癌是一种侵袭性上皮癌，其特点是睾丸核蛋白（nuclear protein in testis，NUT）基因存在重排。它可能起源于中线区域的任何解剖结构，最常见的是鼻窦，其次是肺和纵隔[2]。由于其罕见，这种恶性肿瘤常被排除在临床试验之外，因此唯一可用的证据是病例报告。有报道称纳武利尤单抗为1例NUT肺癌患者带来了长期临床获益[58]。在一项针对3例NUT癌患者的小型研究中，PD-L1表达、TMB、CD8计数和错配修复蛋白表达之间没有明确的相关性[59]。

4 结论

在 SGC 中，一些高级 non-ACC 可能因其免疫激活的 TME 而从免疫治疗中获益。ACC 通常具有类似免疫沙漠的 TME，这可能是其免疫治疗较少产生临床获益的原因。免疫检查点抑制剂与其他靶向治疗的结合可能会增加临床疗效，因此需要进一步的研究。

PNC 对免疫检查点抑制剂的反应与常见的 HNSCC 相似。SNUC 可能从免疫治疗中获益，其与诱导化疗联合治疗局部晚期疾病应在临床试验中进一步评估。ITAC 具有类似免疫沙漠的 TME，因此可能难以从免疫治疗中获益。由于缺乏数据，免疫检查点抑制剂在罕见鼻窦癌（即 NUT 癌、SMARCB1 缺失型癌、ENB）中的作用更加不确定。总而言之，对于 SGC 和鼻窦癌，免疫治疗并非标准治疗，因此不应在临床试验之外实施。

原文符合伦理标准相关声明

Disclosure of Potential Conflicts of Interest Paolo Bossi received fees for consulting or advisory role from Merck, Sanofi, Merck Sharp & Dohme, Sun Pharma, Angelini, Molteni, Bristol-Myers Squibb, and GSK; research funding by GSK, MSD, Sanofi, and BMS.

Lisa Licitra declares the following conflicts of interests: Receipt of grants/research supports (Funds received by my institution for clinical studies and research activities in which I am involved) from AstraZeneca, BMS, Boehringer Ingelheim, Celgene International, Debiopharm International SA, Eisai, Exelixis Inc., Hoffmann-La Roche Ltd., IRX Therapeutics Inc., Medpace Inc., Merck–Serono, MSD, Novartis, Pfizer, and Roche; receipt of honoraria or consultation fees (for public speaking/teaching in medical meetings and/or for expert opinion in advisory boards) from AstraZeneca, Bayer, BMS, Eisai, MSD, Merck–Serono, Boehringer Ingelheim, Novartis, Roche, Debiopharm International SA, Sobi, Ipsen, Incyte Biosciences Italy SRL, Doxa Pharma, Amgen, Nanobiotics Sa, and GSK.

Stefano Cavalieri declares that he has no conflict of interest.

Informed Consent Not applicable for this literature review. Details about ethical approvals and informed consents are provided in each of the cited clinical studies.

参考文献

1. Machiels JP, Leemans CR, Golusinski W et al (2020) Squamous cell carcinoma of the oral cavity, larynx, oropharynx and hypopharynx: EHNS-ESMO-ESTRO clinical practice guidelines for diagnosis, treatment and follow-up. Ann Oncol 31:1462-1475. https://doi.org/10.1016/

j.annonc.2020.07.011
2. El-Naggar AK, Chan JKC, Grandis JR, Takata T, Slootweg PJ (2017) WHO classification of head and neck tumours, 4th edn. WHO-IARC, Lyon
3. RARECARENet—data source and methods. http://www.rarecarenet.eu/. Accessed 20 Sept 2019. Accessed 11 Aug 2021
4. Geiger JL, Ismaila N, Beadle B et al (2021) Management of salivary gland malignancy: ASCO guideline. J Clin Oncol 39:1909-1941. https://doi.org/10.1200/JCO.21.00449
5. Alfieri S, Granata R, Bergamini C et al (2017) Systemic therapy in metastatic salivary gland carcinomas: a pathology-driven paradigm? Oral Oncol 66:58-63. https://doi.org/10.1016/j.oraloncology.2016.12.016
6. Takahashi H, Tada Y, Saotome T et al (2019) Phase II trial of trastuzumab and docetaxel in patients with human epidermal growth factor receptor 2-positive salivary duct carcinoma. J Clin Oncol 37:125-134. https://doi.org/10.1200/JCO.18.00545
7. Ho AS, Kannan K, Roy DM et al (2013) The mutational landscape of adenoid cystic carcinoma. Nat Genet 45:791-798. https://doi.org/10.1038/ng.2643
8. Kurzrock R, Bowles DW, Kang H et al (2020) Targeted therapy for advanced salivary gland carcinoma based on molecular profiling: results from MyPathway, a phase IIa multiple basket study. Ann Oncol 31:412-421. https://doi.org/10.1016/j.annonc.2019.11.018
9. Mosele F, Remon J, Mateo J et al (2020) Recommendations for the use of next-generation sequencing (NGS) for patients with metastatic cancers: a report from the ESMO Precision Medicine Working Group. Ann Oncol 31:1491-1505. https://doi.org/10.1016/J.ANNONC.2020.07.014
10. Shen TK, Teknos TN, Toland AE et al (2014) Salivary gland cancer in BRCA-positive families: a retrospective review. JAMA Otolaryngol Head Neck Surg 140:1213-1217. https://doi.org/10.1001/JAMAOTO.2014.1998
11. Nakano T, Takizawa K, Uezato A et al (2019) Prognostic value of programed death ligand-1 and ligand-2 co-expression in salivary gland carcinomas. Oral Oncol 90:30-37. https://doi.org/10.1016/J.ORALONCOLOGY.2019.01.015
12. Linxweiler M, Kuo F, Katabi N et al (2020) The immune microenvironment and neoantigen landscape of aggressive salivary gland carcinomas differ by subtype. Clin Cancer Res 26:2859-2870. https://doi.org/10.1158/1078-0432. CCR-19-3758
13. Wang F, Xie X, Song M et al (2020) Tumor immune microenvironment and mutational analysis of tracheal adenoid cystic carcinoma. Ann Transl Med. https://doi.org/10.21037/ATM-20-3433
14. Zhou Z, Li M (2021) Evaluation of BRCA1 and BRCA2 as indicators of response to immune checkpoint inhibitors. JAMA Netw Open. https://doi.org/10.1001/JAMANETWORKOPEN.2021.7728
15. Samstein RM, Krishna C, Ma X et al (2021) Mutations in BRCA1 and BRCA2 differentially affect the tumor microenvironment and response to checkpoint blockade immunotherapy. Nat Cancer 1:1188-1203. https://doi.org/10.1038/S43018-020-00139-8
16. Bishop JA, Thompson LDR, Wakely PEJ, Weinreb I (2021) AFIP atlas: tumors of the salivary glands (fifth series), vol 5. ARP Press, Arlington, VA
17. Cavalieri S, Mariani L, Vander Poorten V et al (2020) Prognostic nomogram in patients with metastatic adenoid cystic carcinoma of the salivary glands. Eur J Cancer 136:35-42. https://doi.org/10.1016/J.EJCA.2020.05.013

18. Fujii K, Murase T, Beppu S et al (2017) MYB, MYBL1, MYBL2 and NFIB gene alterations and MYC overexpression in salivary gland adenoid cystic carcinoma. Histopathology 71:823-834. https://doi.org/10.1111/HIS.13281
19. Rettig EM, Tan M, Ling S et al (2015) MYB rearrangement and clinicopathologic characteristics in head and neck adenoid cystic carcinoma. Laryngoscope 125:E292-E299. https://doi.org/10.1002/LARY.25356
20. Ferrarotto R, Mitani Y, Diao L et al (2017) Activating NOTCH1 mutations define a distinct subgroup of patients with adenoid cystic carcinoma who have poor prognosis, propensity to bone and liver metastasis, and potential responsiveness to Notch1 inhibitors. J Clin Oncol 35:352-360. https://doi.org/10.1200/JCO.2016.67.5264
21. Ferrarotto R, Mitani Y, Mcgrail DJ et al (2021) Proteogenomic analysis of salivary adenoid cystic carcinomas defines molecular subtypes and identifies therapeutic targets a C. Clin Cancer Res 27:852-864. https://doi.org/10.1158/1078-0432.CCR-20-1192
22. Sridharan V, Gjini E, Liao X et al (2016) Immune profiling of adenoid cystic carcinoma: PD-L2 expression and associations with tumor-infiltrating lymphocytes. Cancer Immunol Res 4:679-687. https://doi.org/10.1158/2326-6066. CIR-16-0031
23. Mosconi C, de Arruda JAA, de Farias ACR et al (2019) Immune microenvironment and evasion mechanisms in adenoid cystic carcinomas of salivary glands. Oral Oncol 88:95-101. https://doi.org/10.1016/J.ORALONCOLOGY.2018.11.028
24. Kokkali S, Ntokou A, Drizou M et al (2020) Nivolumab in patients with rare head and neck carcinomas: a single center's experience. Oral Oncol 101. https://doi.org/10.1016/J.ORALONCOLOGY.2019.07.002
25. Niwa K, Kawakita D, Nagao T et al (2020) Multicentre, retrospective study of the efficacy and safety of nivolumab for recurrent and metastatic salivary gland carcinoma. Sci Rep. https://doi.org/10.1038/s41598-020-73965-6
26. Rodriguez CP, Wu QV, Voutsinas J et al (2020) A phase II trial of pembrolizumab and vorinostat in recurrent metastatic head and neck squamous cell carcinomas and salivary gland cancer. Clin Cancer Res 26:837-845. https://doi.org/10.1158/1078-0432. CCR-19-2214
27. Fayette J, Even C, Digue L et al (2019) NISCAHN: a phase II, multicenter nonrandomized trial aiming at evaluating nivolumab (N) in two cohorts of patients (pts) with recurrent/metastatic (R/M) salivary gland carcinoma of the head and neck (SGCHN), on behalf of the Unicancer Head & Neck Group. J Clin Oncol. https://doi.org/10.1200/JCO.2019.37.15_SUPPL.6083
28. Tchekmedyian V, Sherman EJ, Dunn L et al (2019) A phase II trial cohort of nivolumab plus ipilimumab in patients (Pts) with recurrent/metastatic adenoid cystic carcinoma (R/M ACC). J Clin Oncol. https://doi.org/10.1200/JCO.2019.37.15_SUPPL.6084
29. Chae YK, Othus M, Patel SP et al (2020) Abstract 3418: a phase II basket trial of dual anti-CTLA-4 and anti-PD-1 blockade in rare tumors (DART) SWOG S1609: the salivary gland tumor cohort. Cancer Res. https://doi.org/10.1158/1538-7445.AM2020-3418
30. Cohen RB, Delord JP, Doi T et al (2018) Pembrolizumab for the treatment of advanced salivary gland carcinoma: findings of the phase 1b KEYNOTE-028 study. Am J Clin Oncol 41:1083-1088. https://doi.org/10.1097/COC.0000000000000429
31. Mahmood U, Bang A, Chen Y et al (2021) A randomized phase 2 study of pembrolizumab with or without radiation in patients with recurrent or metastatic adenoid cystic carcinoma. Int J Radiat Oncol Biol Phys 109:134-144. https://doi.org/10.1016/J.IJROBP.2020.08.018

32. Axitinib and avelumab in treating patients with recurrent or metastatic adenoid cystic carcinoma. Available ClinicalTrials.gov. https://clinicaltrials.gov/ct2/show/NCT03990571. Accessed 11 Aug 2021
33. Lenvatinib and pembrolizumab in people with advanced adenoid cystic carcinoma and other salivary gland cancers. Available ClinicalTrials.gov. https://clinicaltrials.gov/ct2/show/NCT04209660. Accessed 11 Aug 2021
34. Laurie SA, Licitra L (2006) Systemic therapy in the palliative management of advanced salivary gland cancers. J Clin Oncol 24:2673-2678. https://doi.org/10.1200/JCO.2005.05.3025
35. Skálová A, Vanecek T, Sima R et al (2010) Mammary analogue secretory carcinoma of salivary glands, containing the etv6-ntrk3 fusion gene: a hitherto undescribed salivary gland tumor entity. Am J Surg Pathol 34:599-608. https://doi.org/10.1097/PAS.0b013e3181d9efcc
36. Locati LD, Perrone F, Cortelazzi B et al (2016) Clinical activity of androgen deprivation therapy in patients with metastatic/relapsed androgen receptor-positive salivary gland cancers. Head Neck 38:724-731. https://doi.org/10.1002/hed.23940
37. Li BT, Shen R, Offin M et al (2019) Ado-trastuzumab emtansine in patients with HER2 amplified salivary gland cancers (SGCs): results from a phase II basket trial. J Clin Oncol. https://doi.org/10.1200/jco.2019.37.15_suppl.6001
38. Bando H, Kinoshita I, Modi S et al (2021) Trastuzumab deruxtecan (T-DXd) in patients with human epidermal growth factor receptor 2 (HER2)-expressing salivary duct carcinoma: subgroup analysis of two phase 1 studies. J Clin Oncol. https://doi.org/10.1200/JCO.2021.39.15_SUPPL.6079
39. Burman B, Sherman EJ, Dunn L et al (2021) A phase II trial cohort of nivolumab plus ipilimumab in patients (Pts) with recurrent/metastatic salivary gland cancers (R/M SGCs). J Clin Oncol. https://doi.org/10.1200/JCO.2021.39.15_SUPPL.6002
40. Agaimy A, Hartmann A, Antonescu CR et al (2017) SMARCB1 (INI-1)-deficient sinonasal carcinoma: a series of 39 cases expanding the morphologic and clinicopathologic spectrum of a recently described entity. Am J Surg Pathol 41:458-471. https://doi.org/10.1097/PAS.0000000000000797
41. Bishop J, Ogawa T, Stelow E et al (2013) Human papillomavirus-related carcinoma with adenoid cystic-like features: a peculiar variant of head and neck cancer restricted to the sinonasal tract. Am J Surg Pathol 37:836-844. https://doi.org/10.1097/PAS.0B013E31827B1CD6
42. Bishop JA, Andreasen S, Hang JF et al (2017) HPV-related multiphenotypic sinonasal carcinoma: an expanded series of 49 cases of the tumor formerly known as HPV-related carcinoma with adenoid cystic carcinoma-like features. Am J Surg Pathol 41:1690-1701. https://doi.org/10.1097/PAS.0000000000000944
43. Amit M, Abdelmeguid AS, Watcherporn T et al (2019) Induction chemotherapy response as a guide for treatment optimization in sinonasal undifferentiated carcinoma. J Clin Oncol 37:504-512. https://doi.org/10.1200/JCO.18.00353
44. Udager AM, Rolland DCM, McHugh JB et al (2015) High-frequency targetable EGFR mutations in sinonasal squamous cell carcinomas arising from inverted sinonasal papilloma. Cancer Res 75:2600-2606. https://doi.org/10.1158/0008-5472.CAN-15-0340
45. Riobello C, López-Hernández A, Cabal VN et al (2020) IDH2 mutation analysis in undifferentiated and poorly differentiated sinonasal carcinomas for diagnosis and clinical management. Am J Surg Pathol 44:396-405. https://doi.org/10.1097/PAS.0000000000001420

46. Ferris RL, Blumenschein G, Fayette J et al (2016) Nivolumab for recurrent squamous-cell carcinoma of the head and neck. N Engl J Med 375:1856-1867. https://doi.org/10.1056/NEJMoa1602252
47. Cohen EEW, Soulières D, Le Tourneau C et al (2019) Pembrolizumab versus methotrexate, docetaxel, or cetuximab for recurrent or metastatic head-and-neck squamous cell carcinoma (KEYNOTE-040): a randomised, open-label, phase 3 study. Lancet 393:156-167. https://doi.org/10.1016/S0140-6736(18)31999-8
48. Burtness B, Harrington KJ, Greil R et al (2019) Pembrolizumab alone or with chemotherapy versus cetuximab with chemotherapy for recurrent or metastatic squamous cell carcinoma of the head and neck (KEYNOTE-048): a randomised, open-label, phase 3 study. Lancet 394:1915-1928. https://doi.org/10.1016/S0140-6736(19)32591-7
49. Pembrolizumab combined with cetuximab for treatment of recurrent/metastatic head & neck squamous cell carcinoma. Available ClinicalTrials.gov. https://clinicaltrials.gov/ct2/show/NCT03082534. Accessed 11 Aug 2021
50. Denaro N, Merlano M, Numico G et al (2021) Complete response to immunotherapy in sinonasal undifferentiated carcinoma. Tumori. https://doi.org/10.1177/03008916211026971
51. García-Marín R, Reda S, Riobello C et al (2021) Prognostic and therapeutic implications of immune classification by CD8 + tumor-infiltrating lymphocytes and PD-L1 expression in sinonasal squamous cell carcinoma. Int J Mol Sci. https://doi.org/10.3390/IJMS22136926
52. Riobello C, Vivanco B, Reda S et al (2018) Programmed death ligand-1 expression as immunotherapeutic target in sinonasal cancer. Head Neck 40:818-827. https://doi.org/10.1002/HED.25067
53. Bell D, Bell A, Ferrarotto R et al (2020) High-grade sinonasal carcinomas and surveillance of differential expression in immune related transcriptome. Ann Diagn Pathol. https://doi.org/10.1016/J.ANNDIAGPATH.2020.151622
54. De Cecco L, Serafini MS, Facco C et al (2019) A functional gene expression analysis in epithelial sinonasal cancer: biology and clinical relevance behind three histological subtypes. Oral Oncol 90:94-101. https://doi.org/10.1016/j.oraloncology.2019.02.003
55. Bossi P, Perrone F, Miceli R et al (2013) Tp53 status as guide for the management of ethmoid sinus intestinal-type adenocarcinoma. Oral Oncol 49:413-419. https://doi.org/10.1016/J.ORALONCOLOGY.2012.12.011
56. García-Marín R, Reda S, Riobello C et al (2020) CD8 + tumour-infiltrating lymphocytes and tumour microenvironment immune types as biomarkers for immunotherapy in sinonasal intestinal-type adenocarcinoma. Vaccine 8. https://doi.org/10.3390/VACCINES8020202
57. Friedman J, Schumacher JK, Papagiannopoulos P et al (2021) Targeted 595-gene genomic profiling demonstrates low tumor mutational burden in olfactory neuroblastoma. Int Forum Allergy Rhinol 11:58-64. https://doi.org/10.1002/ALR.22595
58. Davis A, Mahar A, Wong K et al (2020) Prolonged disease control on nivolumab for primary pulmonary NUT carcinoma. Clin Lung Cancer. https://doi.org/10.1016/J.CLLC.2020.10.016
59. He M, Chernock R, Zhou S et al (2020) Tumor mutation burden and checkpoint immunotherapy markers in NUT midline carcinoma. Appl Immunohistochem Mol Morphol 28:495-500. https://doi.org/10.1097/PAI.0000000000000781

第9章 头颈部肿瘤免疫治疗预测生物标志物的发展

Development of Predictive Biomarkers to Immunotherapy in Head and Neck Cancer

(Kedar Kirtane, Christine H. Chung 著)

(周亚娟,余笑言,鲁瑛 译)

摘要

免疫治疗已经彻底改变了晚期肿瘤的治疗方式。虽然已经批准免疫治疗用于复发和(或)转移性头颈部肿瘤患者,但仍有很大一部分患者并不能从这一昂贵的治疗中获益,所以发掘预测生物标志物变得尤为重要,以能够准确评估与筛选出更可能从免疫治疗中获益的患者。然而,肿瘤内在和外在因素驱动的免疫抑制和促炎信号之间的相互作用是十分复杂的,所以如果想找到稳定且精准的生物标志物,需要详细了解恶性转化、转移以及抗肿瘤治疗产生的选择压力引起的宿主免疫应答的各个环节。在本章中,我们讨论了免疫治疗耐药的基础知识、有发展前景的免疫治疗预测生物标志物,以及可能有助于优化免疫治疗策略的免疫调节剂的潜在应用。此外,可能需要在多个时间点整合应用多个生物标志物,以最大限度地提高对免疫治疗反应的预测能力。

原作者信息

Kirtane (✉) · C. H. Chung
Moffitt Cancer Center, Tampa, FL, USA
e-mail: Kedar.Kirtane@Moffitt.Org; Christine.Chung@Moffitt.Org

关键词

DNA 修复通路；内源性逆转录病毒；外泌体；头颈部肿瘤；免疫治疗；聚合酶 ε 突变；T 细胞炎性基因表达谱；肿瘤突变负荷；病毒感染

1　引言

除了手术、放疗和化疗之外，免疫治疗也已成为转移性肿瘤患者的主要治疗手段之一。几项开创性研究已经证实，免疫调节是治疗头颈部肿瘤患者的有效方法[1-3]。然而只有少数患者表现出对免疫调节剂的持久反应，因此需要选择合适的患者。临床常发现只有少数患者能从免疫治疗中获益，筛选出能够从免疫治疗中获益的人群是免疫治疗的关键步骤。对于头颈部肿瘤而言，发掘预后生物标志物和预测生物标志物至关重要，对于预后差的转移性肿瘤患者更是如此[4]。预后生物标志物对于风险分层很重要，而预测生物标志物对于获得最大化的治疗效益并使无效治疗的风险最小化也非常重要。要成功发掘生物标志物，需要对肿瘤生物学、治疗药物的作用机制以及耐药机制有深入了解。

2　评估肿瘤内在因素的预测生物标志物

目前的免疫治疗策略主要集中在 T 细胞功能调节上。T 细胞活化需要抗原在抗原呈递细胞（APC）上由主要组织相容性复合体（MHC）呈递到 T 细胞受体（TCR），共刺激分子 CD28 和 B7 通常是 T 细胞激活所必需的。其中的相互作用受到一系列抑制性免疫检查点的严密调控，这些检查点在生理上可以防止对外部或内部攻击产生自身免疫反应[5]。肿瘤细胞常利用这点来下调 T 细胞的反应，否则自身免疫反应会阻止肿瘤的恶性生长和扩散。在这些相互作用中存在大量潜在的生物标志物，可用于评估耐药模式。耐药的潜在生物标志物可能包括肿瘤抗原的缺失和 APC 的抗原递呈缺失，而后者可能由一系列因素引起，包括但不限于抗原递呈机制的改变、β2-微球蛋白的丧失或 MHC 的丧失。在接下来的部分中，我们将讨论能反映引发免疫检查点抑制剂（ICI）敏感性和耐药性的肿瘤内在因素的生物标志物。

2.1 肿瘤突变负荷

肿瘤突变负荷（TMB）指的是肿瘤基因组编码区域每个体细胞突变的总数，其被认为可预测对 ICI 的反应。这在很大程度上反映了这样一种观点：具有较高 TMB 的肿瘤也与较多新抗原相关联，这些新抗原是在肿瘤组织中发现的突变抗原，但在正常细胞中不存在。肿瘤新抗原主要通过 MHC 呈递给 T 细胞，因此在去除免疫检查点抑制后更能够引发免疫反应[6]。值得注意的是，未接受 ICI 治疗的高 TMB 患者的总生存期不如接受 ICI 治疗的患者，这表明 TMB 更适合作为预测对 ICI 疗效的预测生物标志物，而不是简单的预后指标[7]。对于头颈部肿瘤，TMB 截断值为 10.3（即定义为规范化突变负荷的前 20%），其在接受 ICI 治疗时似乎与改善生存相关。

尽管对于接受 ICI 治疗的患者而言，较高的 TMB 和与之相关的较高的新抗原负荷有助于增强免疫识别，但头颈部肿瘤在预示 ICI 反应的基因组特征方面很独特。超过 100 例头颈部肿瘤患者的肿瘤测序数据显示，肿瘤抑制基因中的体细胞移码突变可以预测对 ICI 的反应[8]，在这个队列研究中，病毒介导的头颈部肿瘤和非病毒介导的头颈部肿瘤在反应数量上没有差异。

2.2 烟草暴露和头颈部肿瘤

许多非病毒介导的 HNC 是由于烟草暴露造成的。虽然与吸烟相关的基因特征通常与较高的肿瘤突变负荷相关，但它并不总是与对 ICI 的反应相关。一项使用头颈部肿瘤癌症基因组图谱（The Cancer Genome Atlas, TCGA）测序数据的研究发现，"大量吸烟"的患者总生存率更低[9]。这项研究还表明，吸烟量大与更低水平的免疫浸润、细胞溶解活性和干扰素 γ 信号有关，而与 HPV 状态或头颈部肿瘤的解剖亚位点无关。这与在肺鳞状细胞癌中发现的情况相反，肺鳞状细胞癌对 ICI 反应较强，表明吸烟会因解剖部位和肿瘤微环境（TME）的不同而对肿瘤产生不同影响[10]。对于头颈部肿瘤，吸烟似乎与免疫抑制作用相关，表现为烟草会抑制机体对 ICI 产生强烈免疫反应，而这一免疫反应恰好与细胞溶解活性相关。深入研究发现，吸烟的头颈部肿瘤患者 TME 中 CD8+ 细胞毒性 T 细胞和 PD-L1 阳性细胞数量更少[11]。总之，由于在肿瘤标本中的独特表现，吸烟相关基因特征作为 HNC 中 ICI 反应的预测生物标志物显示出良好前景。

2.3 DNA 修复通路

目前已知 DNA 修复通路的功能异常是肿瘤发生的重要因素之一。例如，同源重组和错配修复的损伤是人类肿瘤的致病性基因组改变[12]。免疫系统与 DNA 修复途径的相互作用在过去十年已成为一个重要领域。直观上，这种联系是合乎逻辑的，DNA 修复通路可以维持基因组稳定性，而这些信号通路的异常可能会导致更高的突变负荷，从而引发免疫反应。

微卫星不稳定性（microsatellite instability, MSI）是 DNA 修复通路出错的结果，导致 DNA 中短的重复序列与最初遗传序列不同。虽然 MSI 经常在各种胃肠道恶性肿瘤中被发现，但在一些头颈部肿瘤中可能也很常见。关于头颈部肿瘤中高 MSI 状态的报道存在显著差异。在一项分析头颈部肿瘤标本的研究中，有 41% 被发现 MSI 水平较高，但其他研究发现的患病率低得多，约为 1%[13-14]。高 MSI 状态作为 ICI 反应的潜在预测生物标志物已被广泛研究，在一项针对转移性肿瘤患者的 II 期研究中，错配修复（mismatch repair, MMR）对 ICI 的临床获益有高度预测性[15]。2017 年，抗 PD-1 药物帕博利珠单抗获得了美国 FDA 的首个泛肿瘤的应用批准，用于治疗高 MSI 的肿瘤患者。

MSI 状态作为预测生物标志物的生物学基础是充分的，因为它通常是 MMR 通路缺陷的结果。MMR 异常与体细胞突变率增加和由此产生的新抗原增加以及炎症介质增加相关联，这些介质可帮助招募细胞毒性 T 细胞[16-17]。尽管高 MSI 头颈部肿瘤患病率可能较低，但其作为预测 ICI 反应的生物标志物可能未来会在临床上应用。

2.4 聚合酶 ε 突变

最近的研究显示缺陷的 DNA 聚合酶活性与肿瘤发生有关[18]。DNA 聚合酶是保证 DNA 复制的高完整性和准确性的关键。特别是 DNA 聚合酶的外切酶活性对于校对不匹配的核苷酸必不可少。近年来的研究表明在多种肿瘤的形成过程中出现了散发的 DNA 聚合酶 ε（POLE）基因突变，包括但不限于子宫内膜癌、胶质母细胞瘤和结直肠癌[19]。POLE 突变往往与高突变负荷和免疫检查点基因的表达升高有关[20]。有一项纳入了 93 名 POLE 基因突变患者的研究发现约 54% 的病例使用帕博利珠单抗后有临床获益[21]。但是，仍然需要进一步研究来证实 POLE 突变是否可以作为 HNC 中 ICI 获益的预测生物标志物。

2.5 人类内源性逆转录病毒

人类内源性逆转录病毒（human endogenous retrovirus, HERV）的去甲基化也有可能提高对免疫治疗的敏感性[22]。HERV 是人类祖先感染逆转录病毒后的 DNA 残留物，在人类基因组中约占 8%[23]。一项使用结直肠癌细胞的研究表明，HERV 的去甲基化可以诱导产生双链 RNA，随后模拟病毒感染并导致对恶性细胞产生先天性和适应性免疫反应[22]。抗病毒反应依赖于Ⅲ型干扰素信号通路的上调，利用免疫系统的力量来消退肿瘤。同样地，使用低剂量去甲基化剂 5-氮胞苷后可使卵巢癌小鼠模型中Ⅰ型干扰素信号通路上调[24]。同样也有数据显示去甲基化药物和 ICI 联用可以使试验中的小鼠存活时间延长，这表明 HERV 的表观遗传学治疗可以刺激上皮肿瘤细胞模型中的抗肿瘤免疫反应。

2.6 人乳头瘤病毒和 EB 病毒

现在普遍认为北美大多数口咽癌与人乳头瘤病毒（HPV）有关[25]。此外，Epstein-Barr 病毒（EBV）感染与鼻咽癌的发病机制显著相关[26]。由于这些肿瘤的发生取决于病毒感染，因此肿瘤细胞可能存在具有肿瘤特异性且为病毒驱动的新抗原，而正常细胞则没有。因此，这些肿瘤特异性靶点可能有助于成为预测生物标志物。

与其他头颈部肿瘤不同，HPV 相关的口咽癌具有独特的流行病学特征。一般来说，受病毒驱动的肿瘤比非病毒驱动的肿瘤对免疫治疗更敏感，因为 CD8+ T 细胞的浸润更多，调节性 T 细胞（Treg）数量更少，并且 PD-L1 表达水平更高[27-28]。但是，关于 HPV 相关 HNC 的 ICI 治疗的大型随机试验中并未显示出 HPV 状态在统计学意义上会影响患者生存[2-3]，这些研究中 HPV 阳性和 HPV 阴性肿瘤的结果类似，表明可能存在一系列复杂多样的机制，这些机制可能与吸烟相关基因特征和新抗原负荷相关[29]。然而，病毒驱动的抗原代表了免疫调节的关键靶点。随着细胞免疫治疗的快速发展，目前还不清楚 TIL 治疗、基因重组 T 细胞受体（TCR）和嵌合抗原受体 T 细胞（CAR T）将如何应用才能够直接靶向这些病毒驱动的致癌蛋白。

2.7 外泌体

外泌体是源自胞内体的膜囊泡，大多数人类细胞都可以分泌。APC 分泌的外泌体富含 MHC Ⅰ和 MHC Ⅱ以及 CD86 等共刺激分子[30]。这些复合物参与免疫系统的呈递，因此是免疫调节的潜在靶点。树突细胞外泌体产生功能性 MHC Ⅰ，能够激活细胞毒性 T 细胞，而肿瘤源性外泌体可以在 APC 之间转移肿瘤特异性抗原并增强抗原特异性免疫应答[30]。尽管外泌体仍处于临床前研究阶段，但在通过基因改造的肿瘤细胞疫苗引发肿瘤抗原特异性 T 细胞反应方面可能发挥作用。

2.8 抗原呈递机制的丢失

抗原呈递机制的改变、β2-微球蛋白（MHC Ⅰ的组成部分）的丢失或 MHC 本身的丢失可能会导致对免疫治疗的耐药。由于免疫治疗的获益取决于肿瘤抗原或新抗原向免疫系统的适当呈递，因此，如果 APC 的丢失是作为既存机制发生的，那么将表现为原发性耐药，如果这种丢失是由于对 ICI 选择性反应而发生的，则表现为获得性耐药[31]。一些过继细胞疗法，特别是基因工程 TCR，已表明免疫编辑导致 APC 关键成分的丢失可成为耐药机制之一。例如，在针对转移性 HPV 相关上皮癌患者中 E7 致癌蛋白的 HPV TCR 中发现了 APC 机制的多种缺陷，包括与抗原处理相关的转运蛋白 1（TAP1）和 TAP2 的丧失、HLA-A*02∶01 中的无义突变，以及 β2-微球蛋白的拷贝数丢失[32]。APC 机制中的类似丢失可以预测对免疫治疗的耐药，因为细胞表面 MHC Ⅰ任何的表达受损都会阻止细胞毒性 T 细胞的充分呈递[33]。

2.9 免疫检查点蛋白的表达

PD-L1 的表达是评估 PD-1 抑制剂敏感性的生物标志物，也是目前研究最充分的预测 ICI 疗效的生物标志物。然而，它仍然不是一个完美的生物标志物，因为免疫治疗有效性的关键是增强对肿瘤细胞的免疫应答，而不是修复肿瘤内信号传导缺陷[34]。此外，不同种类的肿瘤 PD-L1 的表达可能不同。对于头颈部肿瘤，分析 PD-L1 表达最常用的指标是联合阳性评分（CPS）。CPS 是 PD-L1 染色细胞数（即肿瘤内部以及肿瘤微环境中包括淋巴细胞和巨噬细胞在内的细胞）除以总活细胞数，再乘以 100。一般来说，对于头颈部肿瘤，阳性评分意味着 CPS ≥ 1。KEYNOTE-048 研究是一项关于帕博利珠单抗单药或与化疗联合与西妥昔单抗加化疗（EXTREME 方案）疗效对比的随机、开放标签、Ⅲ期研究，其中 CPS ≥ 20 亚组的客观缓解率为 23%，而 CPS ≥ 1 亚组的客观缓解率只有 19%[3]。因为这项研究，帕博利珠单药已经成为复发/转移性头颈部肿瘤的一线标准治疗。但是，PD-L1 在预测头颈部肿瘤疗效方面仍有不足，因为即使是表达水平高的患者使用 ICI 后也有相当大的一部分没有明显获益。此外，目前尚不明确如何在局部晚期头颈部肿瘤患者中应用 ICI 和该生物标志物。JAVELIN 研究表明标准放化疗联合阿维鲁单抗未能明显改善局部晚期头颈部肿瘤患者的生存率[35]。然而，探索性亚组分析显示，CPS ≥ 25 的患者可能在无进展生存方面受益。按照 Bonomo 等（2021）的观点，缺乏关于吸烟的潜在免疫抑制作用的研究以及对放疗和 ICI 间相互作用的理解不足可能导致研究的最终负面结果[36]。

3 评估肿瘤外在因素的预测生物标志物

虽然许多关于免疫治疗生物标志物和耐药性的研究都集中在肿瘤内在因素上，但了解肿瘤细胞与其微环境的复杂相互作用可能对于优化免疫治疗效果至关重要。在本节中，我们将简要回顾肿瘤外在因素，例如 TME 中的一系列免疫细胞和微生物组，这些因素也许可以参与预测免疫治疗反应。

3.1　T 细胞炎症基因表达谱

2017 年，Ayers 等分析了使用帕博利珠单抗治疗的患者基线肿瘤标本的 RNA 基因表达谱（gene expression profile, GEP）[37]，最终确定了一个包含 18 个基因的泛肿瘤 T 细胞炎症基因表达谱，其中包括与抗原呈递、适应性免疫反应和趋化因子表达相关的 IFN-γ 应答基因，其可以辅助预测帕博利珠单抗疗效。另外有一项更大规模的临床试验，纳入了 22 种肿瘤 300 多个使用帕博利珠单抗治疗的患者，旨在评估 T 细胞炎症基因表达谱与 TMB 联合预测免疫治疗的疗效 [38]，结果表明高 GEP 和 TMB 提示帕博利珠单抗疗效更好，而低 GEP 和 TMB 提示帕博利珠单抗疗效更差。这种联合应用生物标志物的模式可能有助于今后为抗 PD-1 治疗的试验设计提供信息，尤其对于头颈部肿瘤。

3.2　调节性 T 细胞和效应 T 细胞

TME 涉及多种细胞并以复杂的方式调节免疫反应，目前已有很多研究评估调节性 T 细胞（Treg）、效应 CD8+ T 细胞（Teff）和髓源性抑制细胞（MDSC）预测不同肿瘤的免疫治疗的疗效。Treg 通常会抑制免疫反应，以防止自身免疫性疾病，并维持自身耐受性，而肿瘤细胞恰恰利用这种机制来逃避宿主免疫系统对肿瘤的破坏。另外，Treg 还可以促进生成肿瘤微环境中的免疫抑制细胞因子，从而使 Teff 难以浸润和破坏肿瘤细胞 [39]，所以通过上调 Treg 来逃避抗肿瘤免疫是肿瘤细胞生存的一种方式，现已发现在某些肿瘤类型中 Treg/Teff 比例较高与较差的预后相关 [40]。理论上如果能有增加 Teff 占比的治疗方法，就可以最大限度地提高免疫治疗的疗效，目前还未研究出这种治疗方法，但不影响这是一个有前景的生物标志物，即高 Treg/Teff 比率表明免疫治疗有效的可能性较低 [39]。

3.3 肿瘤相关巨噬细胞

肿瘤相关巨噬细胞（TAM）也是肿瘤微环境的关键性调节因子。TAM 是一组在肿瘤中发现的终末分化细胞，它们产生免疫抑制细胞因子，促进肿瘤进展[41]。TAM 通过减少 T 细胞增殖所必需的代谢产物，增加炎性细胞因子以及与抑制性受体相互作用激活免疫检查点阻断来抑制 Teff 的作用[41]。TAM 还可以通过促进恶性细胞迁移和内皮内渗透来促进肿瘤向远处转移扩散[42]。因此，TAM 的存在与多个肿瘤的临床预后较差相关[43]。未来的免疫治疗方向可能集中在调节 TAM 在肿瘤微环境中的作用并抑制它们在转移性扩散中的作用。目前 TAM 是作为预后生物标志物应用，驱动耐药性的确切因素仍有待深入研究。

3.4 中性粒细胞与淋巴细胞比值

越来越多的证据表明，中性粒细胞与淋巴细胞比值（neutrophil-lymphocyte ratio, NLR）不仅可以作为全身性炎症反应的指标，还可以作为肿瘤相关炎症的指标，而肿瘤相关炎症在肿瘤的发展和转移中发挥作用[44]。一项对 4000 多名接受免疫治疗的晚期肿瘤患者进行的荟萃分析发现，治疗前较高的中性粒细胞与淋巴细胞比值与较差的总生存期相关[44]，这可能是由于效应性 CD8+ T 细胞对抗肿瘤免疫至关重要，并且促炎症细胞因子也会导致中性粒细胞增加，因此推测 NLR 越高，炎症越严重，特别是在淋巴细胞减少的情况下，可能会抑制宿主的抗肿瘤免疫。对于头颈部肿瘤，放化疗引起的严重治疗相关淋巴细胞减少与疾病进展相关[45]，因此其可能成为头颈部肿瘤强有力的预测生物标志物，不仅可以预测 ICI 疗效，还可以预测疾病进展。

3.5 微生物组

最近有研究表明肠道微生物组可以影响免疫治疗的疗效[46]。Routy 等对肺癌和肾癌的样本进行分析发现，对 ICI 无反应的患者体内的嗜黏蛋白阿克曼菌（Akkermansia muciniphila）水平可能较低。同时还发现与未接受抗生素治疗的患者相比，接受抗生素治疗的患者从 ICI 获益的可能性更小。最后，将已从 ICI 治疗中获益的患者的粪便进行粪菌移植

（microbiota transplantation，FMT），将其移植到接种 MCA-205 肿瘤细胞的小鼠体内，能够改善其对接种后接受 ICI 的疗效，而用同样的方式，将使用 ICI 后没有获益患者的粪便通过 FMT 移植到同样模型的小鼠体内，并未显示有改善疗效的作用。还有研究表明，对接受 ICI 治疗的黑色素瘤患者的口腔和肠道微生物组进行单独分析，观察到获益和不获益患者的细菌多样性和组成存在明显差异[47]。与不获益的患者相比，获益患者可能是因为体内含有更多瘤胃球菌科细菌。随着对 ICI 有反应和无反应患者的相对微生物组群进行更全面的特征分析，FMT 在逆转 ICI 耐药方面的潜力值得期待。

4　整合生物标志物研究的重要性

　　由于免疫治疗反应是多因素的，因此需要在治疗过程中纵向测试多个时间点的多个生物标志物。如前所述，多种生物标志物正在被研究，很可能那些最优的标志物在不同的时间点将联合使用，以预测对免疫治疗的反应。然而，进行充分评估的唯一方法是在不同的空间和时间获取耐药的肿瘤标本。虽然免疫治疗是肿瘤治疗的巨大进步，但目前预测是否获益的方法十分有限，所以需要对这些耐药样本进行大规模分析。

　　此外，随着我们设计出越来越多与分子靶向疗法相结合的联合治疗方案，将免疫治疗生物标志物与其他预测生物标志物整合起来至关重要。例如，第二代测序技术现已广泛应用于临床，用于检测肿瘤、循环系统内的肿瘤细胞和游离 DNA，以及唾液中的基因组和（或）转录组变异[48-50]。对于头颈部肿瘤来说，使用多种预测生物标志物可能对病毒驱动的肿瘤更为重要，因为与非病毒驱动的头颈部肿瘤相比，该类肿瘤具有更多可靶向的致癌突变和导致形成融合蛋白的异位，而非病毒驱动的头颈部肿瘤以及唾液腺恶性肿瘤等罕见肿瘤更可能受益于靶向 HER2 或雄激素受体的治疗[51-53]。利用第二代测序识别各种靶标，并将其与免疫治疗的预测生物标志物整合，有望改善罕见恶性肿瘤患者的生存预后。

5 结论

虽然许多评估免疫治疗疗效的方法正在进行临床试验，但目前 PD-L1 免疫组化是 FDA 唯一批准可用于评估免疫治疗疗效的检测方式，其他方法但都需要前瞻性验证。免疫抑制因子和促炎因子之间存在复杂的相互作用，对于发掘可靠、可行的生物标志物非常重要。此外，宿主免疫反应与恶性转化和扩散的相互作用很复杂，所以单一生物标志物很可能不足以充分预测疗效。在多个时间点整合多种生物标志物将有助于优化对免疫治疗疗效的预测能力。

原文符合伦理标准相关声明

Conflict of Interest Kedar Kirtane declares that he owns stock in Seattle Genetics, Oncternal Therapeutics, and Veru.

Christine H. Chung declares she received honoraria from Bristol-Myers Squibb, Merck, Exelixis, CUE, Sanofi, and Mirati for ad hoc Scientific Advisory Board participation.

Informed Consent Not applicable.

参考文献

1. Ferris RL, Blumenschein G Jr, Fayette J et al (2016) Nivolumab for recurrent squamous-cell carcinoma of the head and neck. N Engl J Med 375:1856-1867. https://doi.org/10.1056/NEJMoa1602252
2. Cohen EE, Soulières D, Le Tourneau C et al (2019) Pembrolizumab versus methotrexate, docetaxel, or cetuximab for recurrent or metastatic head-and-neck squamous cell carcinoma (KEYNOTE-040): a randomised, open-label, phase 3 study. Lancet 393(10167):156-167. https://doi.org/10.1016/S0140-6736(18)31999-8
3. Burtness B, Harrington KJ, Greil R et al (2019) Pembrolizumab alone or with chemotherapy versus cetuximab with chemotherapy for recurrent or metastatic squamous cell carcinoma of the head and neck (KEYNOTE-048): a randomised, open-label, phase 3 study. Lancet 394(10212):1915-1928. https://doi.org/10.1016/S0140-6736(19)32591-7
4. Price KA, Cohen EE (2012) Current treatment options for metastatic head and neck cancer. Curr Treat Options in Oncol 13(1):35-46. https://doi.org/10.1007/s11864-011-0176-y
5. Sharma P, Hu-Lieskovan S, Wargo JA et al (2017) Primary, adaptive, and acquired resistance to cancer immunotherapy. Cell 168(4):707-723. https://doi.org/10.1016/j.cell.2017.01.017
6. Verdegaal EM, De Miranda NF, Visser M et al (2016) Neoantigen landscape dynamics during human melanoma-T cell interactions. Nature 536(7614):91-95. https://doi.org/10.1038/nature18945

7. Samstein RM, Lee C-H, Shoushtari AN et al (2019) Tumor mutational load predicts survival after immunotherapy across multiple cancer types. Nat Genet 51(2):202-206. https://doi.org/10.1038/s41588-018-0312-8
8. Hanna GJ, Lizotte P, Cavanaugh M et al (2018) Frameshift events predict anti-PD-1/L1 response in head and neck cancer. JCI Insight. https://doi.org/10.1172/jci.insight.98811
9. Desrichard A, Kuo F, Chowell D et al (2018) Tobacco smoking-associated alterations in the immune microenvironment of squamous cell carcinomas. J Natl Cancer Inst 110(12):1386-1392. https://doi.org/10.1093/jnci/djy060
10. Rizvi NA, Hellmann MD, Snyder A et al (2015) Mutational landscape determines sensitivity to PD-1 blockade in non-small cell lung cancer. Science 348(6230):124-128. https://doi.org/10.1126/science.aaa1348
11. de la Iglesia JV, Slebos RJ, Martin-Gomez L et al (2020) Effects of tobacco smoking on the tumor immune microenvironment in head and neck squamous cell carcinoma. Clin Cancer Res 26(6):1474-1485. https://doi.org/10.1158/1078-0432.CCR-19-1769
12. Lahtz C, Pfeifer GP (2011) Epigenetic changes of DNA repair genes in cancer. J Mol Cell Biol 3(1):51-58. https://doi.org/10.1093/jmcb/mjq053
13. Demokan S, Suoglu Y, Demir D et al (2006) Microsatellite instability and methylation of the DNA mismatch repair genes in head and neck cancer. Ann Oncol 17(6):995-999. https://doi.org/10.1093/annonc/mdl048
14. Bonneville R, Krook MA, Kautto EA et al (2017) Landscape of microsatellite instability across 39 cancer types. JCO Precis Oncol 1:1-15. https://doi.org/10.1200/PO.17.00073
15. Le DT, Uram JN, Wang H et al (2015) PD-1 blockade in tumors with mismatch-repair deficiency. N Engl J Med 372(26):2509-2520. https://doi.org/10.1056/NEJMoa1500596
16. Boissière-Michot F, Lazennec G, Frugier H et al (2014) Characterization of an adaptive immune response in microsatellite-instable colorectal cancer. Onco Targets Ther. https://doi.org/10.4161/onci.29256
17. Viale G, Trapani D, Curigliano G (2017) Mismatch repair deficiency as a predictive biomarker for immunotherapy efficacy. Biomed Res Int. https://doi.org/10.1155/2017/4719194
18. Church DN, Briggs SE, Palles C et al (2013) DNA polymerase ε and δ exonuclease domain mutations in endometrial cancer. Hum Mol Genet 22(14):2820-2828. https://doi.org/10.1093/hmg/ddt131
19. Rayner E, van Gool IC, Palles C et al (2016) A panoply of errors: polymerase proofreading domain mutations in cancer. Nat Rev Cancer 16(2):71-81. https://doi.org/10.1038/nrc.2015.12
20. Mehnert JM, Panda A, Zhong H et al (2016) Immune activation and response to pembrolizumab in POLE-mutant endometrial cancer. J Clin Invest 126(6):2334-2340. https://doi.org/10.1172/JCI84940
21. Garmezy B, Gheeya JS, Thein KZ et al (2020) Correlation of pathogenic POLE mutations with clinical benefit to immune checkpoint inhibitor therapy. Proc Am Soc Clin Oncol. https://doi.org/10.1200/JCO.2020.38.15_suppl.3008
22. Roulois D, Yau HL, De Carvalho DD (2016) Pharmacological DNA demethylation: implications for cancer immunotherapy. Oncoimmunology. https://doi.org/10.1080/2162402X.2015.1090077
23. Griffiths DJ (2001) Endogenous retroviruses in the human genome sequence. Genome Biol 2(6):1017.1-1017.5. https://doi.org/10.1186/gb-2001-2-6-reviews1017
24. Stone ML, Chiappinelli KB, Li H et al (2017) Epigenetic therapy activates type I interferon

signaling in murine ovarian cancer to reduce immunosuppression and tumor burden. Proc Natl Acad Sci 114(51):E10981-E10990. https://doi.org/10.1073/pnas.1712514114
25. O'Sullivan B, Huang SH, Su J et al (2016) Development and validation of a staging system for HPV-related oropharyngeal cancer by the International Collaboration on Oropharyngeal cancer Network for Staging (ICON-S): a multicentre cohort study. Lancet Oncol 17(4):440-451. https://doi.org/10.1016/S1470-2045(15)00560-4
26. Raghupathy R, Hui EP, Chan ATC (2014) Epstein-Barr virus as a paradigm in nasopharyngeal cancer: from lab to clinic. Am Soc Clin Oncol Educ Book 34(1):149-153. https://doi.org/10.14694/EdBook_AM.2014.34.149
27. Oliva M, Spreafico A, Taberna M et al (2019) Immune biomarkers of response to immune-checkpoint inhibitors in head and neck squamous cell carcinoma. Ann Oncol 30(1):57-67. https://doi.org/10.1093/annonc/mdy507
28. Matlung SE, Wilhelmina van Kempen PM, Bovenschen N et al (2016) Differences in T-cell infiltrates and survival between HPV+ and HPV-oropharyngeal squamous cell carcinoma. Future Sci OA. https://doi.org/10.4155/fso.15.88
29. Shamseddine AA, Burman B, Lee NY et al (2021) Tumor immunity and immunotherapy for HPV-related cancers. Cancer Discov. https://doi.org/10.1158/2159-8290.CD-20-1760
30. Chaput N, Taïeb J, Schartz NE et al (2004) Exosome-based immunotherapy. Cancer Immunol Immunother 53(3):234-239. https://doi.org/10.1007/s00262-003-0472-x
31. Iorgulescu JB, Braun D, Oliveira G et al (2018) Acquired mechanisms of immune escape in cancer following immunotherapy. Genome Med 10(1):1-4. https://doi.org/10.1186/s13073-018-0598-2
32. Nagarsheth NB, Norberg SM, Sinkoe AL et al (2021) TCR-engineered T cells targeting E7 for patients with metastatic HPV-associated epithelial cancers. Nat Med 27(3):419-425. https://doi.org/10.1038/s41591-020-01225-1
33. Jenkins RW, Barbie DA, Flaherty KT (2018) Mechanisms of resistance to immune checkpoint inhibitors. Br J Cancer 118(1):9-16. https://doi.org/10.1038/bjc.2017.434
34. Patel SP, Kurzrock R (2015) PD-L1 expression as a predictive biomarker in cancer immunotherapy.Mol Cancer Ther 14(4):847-856. https://doi.org/10.1158/1535-7163.MCT-14-0983
35. Lee NY, Ferris RL, Psyrri A et al (2021) Avelumab plus standard-of-care chemoradiotherapy versus chemoradiotherapy alone in patients with locally advanced squamous cell carcinoma of the head and neck: a randomised, double-blind, placebo-controlled,multicentre, phase 3 trial. Lancet Oncol 22(4):450-462. https://doi.org/10.1016/S1470-2045(20)30737-3
36. Bonomo P, Orlandi E, Bossi P (2021) Patient selection for immunotherapy in head and neck cancer. Lancet Oncol. https://doi.org/10.1016/S1470-2045(21)00237-0
37. Ayers M, Lunceford J, Nebozhyn M et al (2017) IFN-γ-related mRNA profile predicts clinical response to PD-1 blockade. J Clin Invest 127(8):2930-2940. https://doi.org/10.1172/JCI91190
38. Cristescu R, Mogg R, Ayers M et al (2018) Pan-tumor genomic biomarkers for PD-1 checkpoint blockade-based immunotherapy. Science. https://doi.org/10.1126/science.aar3593
39. Murciano-Goroff YR, Warner AB, Wolchok JD (2020) The future of cancer immunotherapy: microenvironment-targeting combinations. Cell Res 30(6):507-519. https://doi.org/10.1038/s41422-020-0337-2
40. Preston CC, Maurer MJ, Oberg AL et al (2013) The ratios of CD8+ T cells to CD4+ CD25+

FOXP3+ and FOXP3-T cells correlate with poor clinical outcome in human serous ovarian cancer. PLoS One. https://doi.org/10.1371/journal.pone.0080063
41. Petty AJ, Yang Y (2017) Tumor-associated macrophages: implications in cancer immunotherapy. Immunotherapy 9(3):289-302. https://doi.org/10.2217/imt-2016-0135
42. Bonde A-K, Tischler V, Kumar S et al (2012) Intratumoral macrophages contribute to epithelial-mesenchymal transition in solid tumors. BMC Cancer 12(1):1-15. https://doi.org/10.1186/1471-2407-12-35
43. Qian B-Z, Pollard JW (2010) Macrophage diversity enhances tumor progression and metastasis. Cell 141(1):39-51. https://doi.org/10.1016/j.cell.2010.03.014
44. Jiang T, Qiao M, Zhao C et al (2018) Pretreatment neutrophil-to-lymphocyte ratio is associated with outcome of advanced-stage cancer patients treated with immunotherapy: a meta-analysis. Cancer Immunol Immunother 67(5):713-727. https://doi.org/10.1007/s00262-018-2126-z
45. Campian JL, Sarai G, Ye X et al (2014) Association between severe treatment-related lymphopenia and progression-free survival in patients with newly diagnosed squamous cell head and neck cancer. Head Neck 36(12):1747-1753. https://doi.org/10.1002/hed.23535
46. Routy B, Le Chatelier E, Derosa L et al (2018) Gut microbiome influences efficacy of PD-1-based immunotherapy against epithelial tumors. Science 359(6371):91-97. https://doi.org/10.1126/science.aan3706
47. Gopalakrishnan V, Spencer CN, Nezi L et al (2018) Gut microbiome modulates response to anti-PD-1 immunotherapy in melanoma patients. Science 359(6371):97-103. https://doi.org/10.1126/science.aan4236
48. Bettegowda C, Sausen M, Leary RJ et al (2014) Detection of circulating tumor DNA in early- and late-stage human malignancies. Sci Transl Med. https://doi.org/10.1126/scitranslmed.3007094
49. Diaz LA Jr, Bardelli A (2014) Liquid biopsies: genotyping circulating tumor DNA. J Clin Oncol 32(6):579-586. https://doi.org/10.1200/JCO.2012.45.2011
50. Wang Y, Springer S, Mulvey CL et al (2015) Detection of somatic mutations and HPV in the saliva and plasma of patients with head and neck squamous cell carcinomas. Sci Transl Med. https://doi.org/10.1126/scitranslmed.aaa8507
51. Haddad R, Colevas AD, Krane JF et al (2003) Herceptin in patients with advanced or metastatic salivary gland carcinomas. A phase II study. Oral Oncol 39(7):724-727. https://doi.org/10.1016/s1368-8375(03)00097-6
52. Fushimi C, Tada Y, Takahashi H et al (2018) A prospective phase II study of combined androgen blockade in patients with androgen receptor-positive metastatic or locally advanced unresectable salivary gland carcinoma. Ann Oncol 29(4):979-984. https://doi.org/10.1093/annonc/mdx771
53. Cancer Genome Atlas Network (2015) Comprehensive genomic characterization of head and neck squamous cell carcinomas. Nature 517(7536):576-582. https://doi.org/10.1038/nature14129

专业术语缩略语表

缩写	英文全称	中文全称
Ab	antibody	抗体
ACC	adenoid cystic carcinoma	腺样囊性癌
Ag	antigen	抗原
AJCC	American Joint Committee on Cancer	美国癌症联合委员会
APC	antigen presenting cell	抗原呈递细胞
APM	antigen processing machinery	抗原加工元件
AR	androgen receptor	雄激素受体
CI	confidence interval	置信区间
CPS	combined positive score	联合阳性评分
CR	complete response	完全缓解
CRT	chemoradiotherapy	化放疗
CTL	cytotoxic T lymphocyte	细胞毒性 T 细胞
CTLA-4	cytotoxic T lymphocyte-associated antigen 4	细胞毒性 T 淋巴细胞相关抗原 4
DAMP	damage-associated molecular pattern	损伤相关分子模式
DC	dendritic cell	树突细胞
DCR	disease control rate	疾病控制率
DFS	disease-free survival	无病生存期，无病生存率
DOR	duration of response	缓解持续时间
EBNA	Epstein-Barr nuclear antigen	Epstein-Barr 核抗原
EBV	Epstein-Barr virus	EB 病毒
EGFR	epidermal growth factor receptor	表皮生长因子受体
EMA	European Medicines Agency	欧洲药品管理局
ENB	esthesioneuroblastoma	嗅神经母细胞瘤

缩写	英文全称	中文全称
ER	endoplasmic reticulum	内质网
ESMO	European Society for Medical Oncology	欧洲肿瘤内科学会
EXTREME	platinum-5-FU-cetuximab	铂类、氟尿嘧啶（5-FU）、西妥昔单抗联用
FDA	U.S. Food and Drug Administration	美国食品药品监督管理局
FGL	fibrinogen-like protein	纤维蛋白原样蛋白
GAL	galectin	半乳凝素
GAS	gamma-activated sequence	γ活化序列
GEP	gene expression profile	基因表达谱
GHS	global health status	整体健康状态
GITR	glucocorticoid-induced TNFR family-related gene	糖皮质激素诱导的TNFR相关基因
GM-CSF	granulocyte-macrophage colony-stimulating factor	粒细胞-巨噬细胞集落刺激因子
HDAC	histone deacetylase	组蛋白去乙酰化酶
HER2	human epidermal growth factor receptor 2	人表皮生长因子受体2
HERV	human endogenous retrovirus	人类内源性逆转录病毒
HLA	human leukocyte antigen	人类白细胞抗原
HMGB1	high mobility group box protein 1	高迁移率族蛋白B1
HNC	head and neck cancer	头颈部肿瘤
HNSCC	squamous cell cancer of the head and neck	头颈部鳞状细胞癌
HPD	hyperprogressive disease	超进展性疾病
HPV	human papillomavirus	人乳头瘤病毒
HR	hazard ratio	风险比
ICB	immune checkpoint blockade	免疫检查点阻断
IC	investigator's choice	研究者选择
ICI	immune checkpoint inhibitor	免疫检查点抑制剂
ICOS	inducible T cell co-stimulator	诱导性共刺激分子

缩写	英文全称	中文全称
ICOS-L	inducible T cell co-stimulator ligand	诱导性共刺激分子配体
IFN-γ	interferon gamma	干扰素 γ
IL	interleukin	白介素
IMRT	intensity-modulated RT	调强放疗
IO	immunotherapy	免疫治疗
irAE	immune-related adverse event	免疫相关不良事件
irPRC	immune-related pathologic response criteria	免疫相关病理反应标准
irRC	immune-related response criteria	免疫相关反应标准
irRECIST	immune-related Response Evaluation Criteria in Solid Tumors	实体瘤免疫相关疗效评价标准
ITAM	immunoreceptor tyrosine-based activation motif	免疫受体酪氨酸基激活基序
ITIFS	immunoreceptor tyrosine-based inhibitory motif	免疫受体酪氨酸基抑制基序
ITT	intent to treat population	意向性治疗人群
JAK2	Janus kinase 2	Janus 激酶 2
LA-NPC	locally advanced nasopharyngeal carcinoma	局部晚期鼻咽癌
LAG-3	lymphocyte activation gene-3	淋巴细胞活化基因 3
LMP	latent membrane protein	潜伏膜蛋白
LSECtin	liver and lymph node sinusoidal endothelial cell C-type lectin	肝和淋巴结窦状内皮细胞 C 型凝集素
MDSC	myeloid-derived suppressor cell	髓源性抑制细胞
MHC	major histocompatibility complex	主要组织相容性复合体
MMR	mismatch repair	错配修复
MPR	major pathologic response	主要病理学缓解
MSI	microsatellite instability	微卫星不稳定性
MTD	maximum tolerated dose	最大耐受剂量
NA, N/A	not applicable	不适用
NCCN	National Comprehensive Cancer Network	美国国家综合癌症网络

缩写	英文全称	中文全称
NK	natural killer	自然杀伤
NLR	neutrophil-to-lymphocyte ratio	中性粒细胞与淋巴细胞比值
NLRC5	caspase recruitment domain containing 5	半胱天冬酶招募结构域 5
NPC	nasopharyngeal cancer	鼻咽癌
NPR	no pathologic response	无病理学缓解
NR	not reached	未达到
NUT	nuclear protein in testis	睾丸核蛋白
OPC	oropharyngeal cancer	口咽癌
OPSCC	oropharyngeal squamous cell carcinoma	口咽鳞状细胞癌
ORR	overall response rate, objective response rate	总缓解率，客观缓解率
OS	overall survival	总生存期，总生存率
PAMP	pathogen-associated molecular pattern	病原体相关分子模式
pCR	pathologic complete response	病理学完全缓解
PD-1	programmed cell death receptor 1	程序性死亡受体 1
PD-L1	programmed cell death ligand 1	程序性死亡受体配体 1
PFS	progression-free survival	无进展生存期，无进展生存率
PGE2	prostaglandin E2	前列腺素 E2
PNC	paranasal sinus carcinomas	鼻腔鼻窦癌
PPR	partial pathologic response	部分病理学缓解
PR	partial response	部分缓解
pTR	pathologic tumor response	病理学肿瘤缓解
QoL	quality of life	生活质量
R/M	recurrent/metastatic	复发和（或）转移性，复发/转移性
RT	radiotherapy	放射治疗，放疗
SCC	squamous cell cancer	鳞状细胞癌
SGC	salivary gland carcinoma	唾液腺癌
SHP2	Src homology domain-containing phosphatase 2	含 Src 同源结构域的磷酸酶 2

缩写	英文全称	中文全称
SITC	The Society for Immunotherapy of Cancer	美国癌症免疫治疗学会
STAT1	signal transducer and activator of transcription 1	信号转导及转录激活因子 1
TAA	tumor-associated antigen	肿瘤相关抗原
TAM	tumor-associated macrophage	肿瘤相关巨噬细胞
TAP	transporter associated with antigen processing	抗原加工相关转运蛋白
Tapasin	TAP-associated protein	TAP 相关蛋白
TCGA	The Cancer Genome Atlas	癌症基因组图谱
TCR	T cell receptor	T 细胞受体
Teff	effector T cell	效应 T 细胞
TGF-β	transforming growth factor beta	转化生长因子 -β
TIGIT	T cell immunoglobulin and immunoreceptor tyrosine-based inhibitory motif	T 细胞免疫球蛋白及免疫受体酪氨酸基抑制基序
TIL	tumor-infiltrating lymphocyte	肿瘤浸润性淋巴细胞
TIM-3	T cell immunoglobulin mucin-3	T 细胞免疫球蛋白黏蛋白 3
TMB	tumor mutational burden	肿瘤突变负荷
TME	tumor microenvironment	肿瘤微环境
TNFR	tumor necrosis factor receptor	肿瘤坏死因子受体
TNFRSF	tumor necrosis factor receptor superfamily	肿瘤坏死因子受体超家族
TORS	transoral robotic surgery	经口机器人手术
TPS	tumor proportion score	肿瘤比例评分
TRAE	treatment-related adverse event	治疗相关不良事件
TRAF-3	TNF receptor-associated factor 3	肿瘤坏死因子受体相关因子 3
Treg	regulatory T cell	调节性 T 细胞
VISTA	V-domain Ig suppressor of T cell activation	T 细胞活化的 V 结构域 Ig 抑制因子
β2M	beta-2-microglobulin	β2- 微球蛋白